Understanding Menopause

KAREN BALLARD

WILEY

Other Wiley Editorial Offices

John Wiley & Sons Inc., 111 River Street, Hoboken, NJ 07030, USA

Jossey-Bass, 989 Market Street, San Francisco, CA 94103-1741, USA

Wiley-VCH Verlag GmbH, Boschstr. 12, D-69469 Weinheim, Germany

John Wiley & Sons Australia Ltd, 33 Park Road, Milton, Queensland 4064, Australia

John Wiley & Sons (Asia) Pte Ltd, 2 Clementi Loop #02-01, Jin Xing Distripark, Singapore 129809

John Wiley & Sons Canada Ltd, 22 Worcester Road, Etobicoke, Ontario, Canada M9W 1L1

Wiley also publishes its books in a variety of electronic formats. Some content that appears in print may not be available in electronic books.

Library of Congress Cataloging-in-Publication Data

Ballard, Karen, 1962–
   Understanding menopause / Karen Ballard.
       p. ; cm. – (Understanding illness & health)
Includes index.
   ISBN 0-470-84471-X (alk. paper)
1. Menopause – Popular works.
   [DNLM: 1. Menopause. 2. Estrogen Replacement Therapy. WP 580 B189u
2003]   I. Title. II. Series.
   RG186 .B337 2003
   618.1′75 – dc21

                                 2002153125

British Library Cataloguing in Publication Data

A catalogue record for this book is available from the British Library

ISBN 0-470-84471-X

Illustrations by Elizabeth Anne Harri

Typeset in 9.5/13pt Photina by Laserwords Private Limited, Chennai, India
Printed and bound in Great Britain by TJ International Ltd, Padstow, Cornwall
This book is printed on acid-free paper responsibly manufactured from sustainable forestry in which at least two trees are planted for each one used for paper production.

Understanding
Menopause

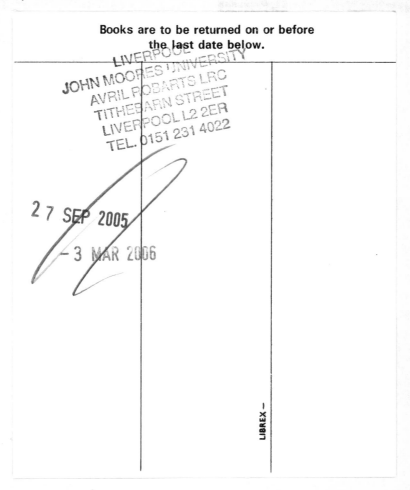

**Books are to be returned on or before
the last date below.**

Understanding Illness and Health

Many health problems and worries are strongly influenced by our thoughts and feelings. These exciting new books, written by experts in the psychology of health, are essential reading for sufferers, their families and friends.

Each book presents objective, easily understood information and advice about what the problem is, the treatments available and, most importantly, how your state of mind can help or hinder the way you cope. You will discover how to have a positive, hopeful outlook, which will help you choose the most effective treatment for you and your particular lifestyle, with confidence.

The series is edited by JANE OGDEN, Reader in Health Psychology, Guy's, King's and St Thomas' School of Medicine, King's College London, UK

Titles in the series

Contents

About the author

KAREN BALLARD is a medical sociologist with a particular interest in women's health issues. She has carried out extensive research into women's experiences of the menopause and their use of hormone replacement therapy, and has recently had a series of papers in this area of work accepted for publication. She is an academic at King's College London, where she works in the department of General Practice and Primary Care.

Acknowledgements

Many people have provided me with advice and encouragement along the course of writing this book, and to them I am very grateful. I would like to say a special thank you to all of the women who participated in the *Women's Health Study*, without whom this book would not have been possible.

Introduction

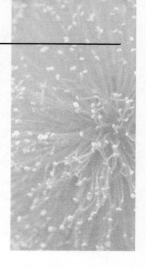

The word 'menopause' originates from the Greek words *menos* (month) and *pausos* (ending), and simply means the cessation of monthly menstruation, although the term menopause was not used by doctors until 1821. Today, on average, the menopause occurs naturally at the age of 51 years, although many women cease to menstruate a few years before or after this age. Eighty per cent of women will have reached the menopause by the age of 54 years.

There are two other terms, the 'climacteric' and the 'change of life', which are also frequently used to describe changes associated with the menopause. Climacteric is also from the Greek language and represents the steps of a ladder, which, it has been suggested, reflects the passage to a different stage in a woman's life. The climacteric refers to the period of time during which changes to the ovary occur. These changes result in a diminishing reproductive function, which is finally lost around the time of the menopause. Changes in the ovary start around 10–15 years before the menopause and continue for around five years after the cessation of menstruation.

In addition to these biological changes, there are a number of social and emotional changes that may also arise at the time of the menopause. Changes in employment, becoming a carer for elderly relatives, changes in relationships with children, and also in body image, may all contribute to an altered outlook on life. The term, 'change of life' represents all of these biological, emotional and social changes. In this way the menopause occurs as part of the wider experience of the change of life. Within this book, the biological, emotional and social changes will be discussed.

The menopause is not a new phenomenon. Indeed, doctors in the ancient world, such as Hippocrates (*circa* 460–377 BC) described the cessation of menstruation as something that happened to all women around the age of 40 years. There has been, however, a significant change in medical explanations about the cause of the menopause, and the symptoms that are likely to be experienced. For example, prior to the nineteenth century, it was generally believed that the menopause was caused by blood becoming trapped within the body.

Like women of today, in the past women experienced symptoms to varying degrees, with some reporting hardly any changes, or none at all, and others reporting quite severe symptoms. Since menstruation was thought to be the body's natural way of cleansing itself, symptoms such as hot flushes were thought to be due to the toxic effects of having blood trapped in the body. Treatments at that time, therefore, focused almost entirely on getting this 'trapped' blood out of the body. Women often had to endure treatments such as having leeches placed on the cervix to draw out the blood directly from the womb.

Once knowledge about the ovaries increased, however, scientists were able to show that the menopause followed a decrease in the production of female hormones. Initially, female hormones were replaced by using desiccated animal ovaries. Once the female hormone oestrogen was identified, however, it became possible to develop more effective and acceptable treatments. The first synthetic preparations of hormone replacement therapy (HRT) became available in the 1930s and, since this time, there has been a huge growth in the number of different preparations available. Today, there are over fifty different types of HRT.

As more and more women use HRT, research has been carried out to try and determine the pros and cons of the therapy. Not all the results, however, have been consistent. For example, some studies report that HRT protects women against heart disease, whilst others have shown that it increases the risk of heart problems. In addition, early studies indicated that HRT did not increase the risk of breast cancer, whereas recent studies have reported a slight increased risk when the therapy is taken for over 4 years.

These apparently contradictory results have largely arisen because of differences, and often inadequacies, in the study design. In addition, many studies have counted all users of HRT as one group, despite variations in the dose or duration of use, or in the type of HRT being used. Thus, it is possible that certain types of HRT, when taken at a specific dose, may be more protective (or harmful) than other types and doses of HRT.

When interpreting research results, it is particularly important to recognise that some HRT preparations only contain the female hormone, oestrogen, whilst others contain both oestrogen plus another female hormone, progesterone. Women who have not had a hysterectomy need to take progesterone in order to protect them against the risk of endometrial cancer (cancer of the lining of the womb). In addition to these differences, some HRT preparations provide progesterone continuously, while others require it to be taken at the end of the cycle only.

Although in recent years there have been moves to encourage women to be involved in decisions about hormone replacement therapy, the conflicting messages arising from much of the research can leave women uncertain about what to do. It is probably not surprising, therefore, that there has been a re-emergence in the use of alternative treatments for the menopause. Women have taken herbal remedies in order to help relieve menopausal symptoms for many centuries. The effectiveness of these treatments, however, is largely unknown. This does not mean that they are not effective, but rather that they have not been subjected to rigorous research in the same way that HRT has. Research into the effectiveness of any treatment is costly and, while the pharmaceutical industry has funded much of the research into HRT, few organisations have been willing to fund large-scale studies into alternative treatments. This situation, however, is changing and recent research has shown that certain alternative treatments are effective for use during the menopause.

The aims of this book are twofold. Firstly, it aims to provide up-to-date information about the biological changes that occur during the menopause and, where appropriate, to discuss the treatment options available to women. There are clearly a number of mixed messages being reported about many of the treatments used during the menopause, and a key aim of this book is to try and clarify the research results. In addition to biological changes, the menopause can also be a time of many social changes, with alterations in work and home circumstances occurring alongside possible changes in body image and self-identity. The second aim of this book is, therefore, to explore women's experiences of the biological and social changes associated with the menopause. To do this, the book draws on the *Women's Health Study*.

The *Women's Health Study*

The *Women's Health Study* was carried out during the years 1999 and 2000, in two stages. The first stage consisted of a postal survey sent to 650 women aged 51 to 57 years, and the second stage involved in-depth interviews with 32 of these women, who were asked to discuss their experiences of the menopause and their use of treatments. The women varied in terms of their experiences of menopausal symptoms, whether they had had a hysterectomy, had taken HRT or alternative therapies, and social class.

Within the book, you will see quotes from women's discussions during the interview, which should bring the experiences of the women to life and add meaning to the information that is being given. All names and any identifying details, however, have been changed. I have tried to weave women's accounts of their experiences in between medical information and advice about the menopause. The purpose of doing this is to make the book more personal. One of the things that women frequently expressed at interview was a need to know whether their experiences were normal. As will become apparent throughout the book, defining 'normal menopause' is not such an easy task. Nevertheless, I hope that it will be possible for women to see that they are not alone in their experiences.

The structure of this book

In addition to this introduction, the book has a total of 10 chapters. Although you may wish to read each chapter in turn, it is not necessary to do this. While the chapters are all linked to each other, they are written in a way that allows each chapter, or section of a chapter, to be read separately. Some aspects of the book, such as the chapter on the history of the menopause and treatments (Chapter 6), are written purely for your interest, whereas others, such as the chapter on experiencing symptoms (Chapter 2), have a more practical application.

Chapter 1 focuses largely on the biological changes that occur before, during and after the menopause, outlining the changes during the normal menstrual cycle, as well as those associated with the menopause. Having discussed these hormone-induced changes, the chapter ends by outlining the impact of a reduction in oestrogen on different parts of the body.

Since most women experience some symptoms that they associate with the menopause, Chapter 2 not only outlines the most frequently reported symptoms, but also provides a guide for treatment options. Possible treatments in the form of self-help, alternative therapies and conventional medicines are outlined. Also in this chapter, the survey and interview results from the *Women's Health Study* are used to illustrate the extent to which women experience symptoms, as well as the impact that the symptoms may have on their lives.

Prior to the menopause, many women have bleeding problems, often experiencing either irregular or heavy periods. Although some women find that they are able to cope with an increased heaviness in menstruation, others may find it necessary to consider treatment options. Chapter 3 describes both medical and surgical treatments for heavy bleeding, outlining the different types of hysterectomy that are performed, as well as newer procedures such as endometrial ablation.

Although much of the focus in the first chapters of the book is on the biological changes relating to the menopause, Chapter 4 focuses on the social changes that often occur during the middle years. Using the interviews with women from the *Women's Health Study*, women's experiences of a number of social changes, such as becoming a carer for elderly relatives, changes in employment, and changes in body image, are described.

Since there has been an increased interest in the long-term effects of the menopause on women's health, Chapter 5 discusses three diseases that appear to be influenced by oestrogen levels: osteoporosis (brittle bone disease), heart disease, and Alzheimer's disease. In addition to describing how these conditions arise, potential risk factors for the three diseases are outlined, along with ways in which women can help to reduce their risks.

Having discussed the modern-day ways of thinking about and experiencing the menopause, Chapter 6 describes how things have changed over time. Starting from as far back as the eleventh century and ending with current-day thinking, developments in medicine and the way in which the menopause is managed are explored.

Chapter 7 discusses the different types of non-hormonal treatments used for the menopause, outlining where there is evidence to support the claims for their effectiveness. Once more, interviews with women from the *Women's Health Study* are used to explore personal experiences of using non-hormonal preparations.

Chapter 8 discusses the main types of hormonal treatments used during and after the menopause. In addition to outlining the various types of HRT, such as 'synthetic' and 'natural' preparations, the different routes that they can be taken is discussed. The *Women's Health Study* survey is also used to illustrate the number of women taking HRT and the reasons why they choose to do so. The risks associated with taking HRT, as well as the contra-indications for use is discussed in detail.

Since many women express concerns about the need for contraception during and after the menopause, Chapter 9 discusses the risk of pregnancy after the menopause and outlines different contraception options.

Chapter 10 considers future developments in understanding the menopause. Here, the changing emphasis, within the Western world, on lifestyle and health risk is discussed in the context of the menopause. In addition, ongoing developments in treatments for the menopause are outlined. Following Chapter 10, there is a list of contact details for various organisations which provide further information and support for women going through the menopause.

Biological changes during the menopause

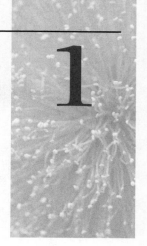

This chapter focuses on the biological changes that occur prior to, during and after the menopause. To help understand these changes the structure of the female reproductive organs and the process of normal menstruation is firstly outlined.

The female reproductive organs

The female reproductive system comprises the uterus (or womb), two ovaries connected to the uterus by fallopian tubes, and the vagina. Figure 1.1 shows the position of these organs.

The uterus is a muscular organ shaped like a pear. It is about $7\frac{1}{2}$ cm long and 5 cm wide, but is able to stretch during pregnancy as the baby grows. The lining of the uterus, called the endometrium, contains numerous blood vessels, which provide nourishment for the growing baby. When a woman is not pregnant, menstruation occurs as the endometrium is shed. The cervix is the lower part of the uterus and connects to the vagina.

The two tubes leaving the uterus are called the fallopian tubes, each being about 10 cm long. These tubes provide a connection between the ovaries and the uterus so that the egg (ovum) can be transported to the uterus for implantation. The ovaries are the female sex glands and sit on either side of the uterus. They contain millions of ovarian follicles and each month one of these follicles matures to produce an egg. The ovaries also produce the female hormones, oestrogen and progesterone, and the male hormones, testosterone and androstenedione.

The menstrual cycle

From puberty to the menopause, women experience a series of menstrual cycles, each occurring approximately every 28 days. During each cycle a sequence of bodily changes occur. The menstrual cycle is divided into three phases:

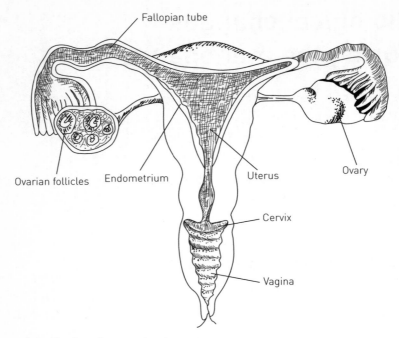

Figure 1.1. The female reproductive system.

(1) The follicular phase – during this phase, follicle-stimulating hormone (FSH), which is produced by the pituitary gland (situated beneath the base of the brain) stimulates the growth of several ovarian follicles. Generally, just one follicle matures and contains an ovum (egg). As the follicle grows, it produces the hormone oestrogen, which stimulates the lining of the womb to thicken. Once the ovarian follicle has reached maturity, it ruptures (ovulation) and the ovum is released. The follicle then stops producing any more oestrogen and, in turn, the lining of the womb ceases to get any thicker.

(2) The luteal phase – after ovulation what remains of the ovarian follicle is stimulated by a hormone called luteinising hormone to develop the corpus luteum. The corpus luteum then produces the hormones, progesterone and oestrogen, which stimulate the lining of the womb to produce a watery fluid that helps the sperm to swim towards the fallopian tubes for fertilisation. If fertilisation does not occur, the next phase of the cycle begins.

(3) The menstrual phase – if fertilisation of the egg does not occur, the production of luteinising hormone ceases, and the corpus luteum breaks down. In turn, the production of progesterone and oestrogen decreases and the lining of the womb breaks down, leading to menstruation.

The ovarian hormones

The ovaries produce both female and male hormones. The main female hormones are oestrogen and progesterone and the main male hormones are testosterone and androstenedione.

Oestrogen

There are two types of oestrogen, oestradiol and oestrone. Oestradiol is the main source of oestrogen for women up until the time of the menopause, and is produced by the ovaries. From puberty to around the age of 30, the levels of oestradiol reach their highest (average blood levels of 450 to 550 pmol/l). After around the age of 30 years the production of oestradiol gradually lessens. A few years before the menopause, oestradiol blood levels are around 200–300 pmol/l. After the menopause, however, levels of oestradiol fall to around 80 pmol/l.

The other source of oestrogen (oestrone) comes from the adrenal glands, which sit on the top of each kidney. These glands produce a male hormone called androstenedione, which is converted in the fatty tissue to an oestrogen called oestrone. The average level of oestrone after the menopause is around 100 pmol/l. Since the conversion of androstenedione takes place in the fatty tissue, women with greater amounts of fatty tissue produce higher levels of oestrone.

The main functions of oestrogen are to:

- Help regulate menstruation.
- Help prepare the body for fertilisation.
- Stimulate the lining of the womb so that it thickens.
- Maintain lubrication of the vagina.
- Help maintain the acid level in the vagina, thereby protecting against infections.
- Work in conjunction with progesterone to help with the breakdown of the endometrium (lining of the womb) in the second stage of the menstrual cycle.
- Maintain a supply of calcium to the bones.
- Help maintain the health of blood vessel walls.
- Reduce the blood cholesterol level.
- Bring about the development of secondary sex characteristics, i.e. the breasts and nipples.
- Influence body shape at puberty, resulting in women having broader hips and narrower shoulders than men, and a tendency to deposit fat on the hips and thighs.

- Increase elasticity of the skin.
- Influence the growth of body hair, so that women have less body hair and more scalp hair than men.
- Stop the growth of the arm and leg bones, resulting in women being generally shorter than men.

Progesterone

The ovaries provide the only source of progesterone, where it is produced after ovulation.

The main functions of progesterone are to:

- Help prepare the body for fertilisation and maintain pregnancy.
- Work in conjunction with oestrogen, to help with the breakdown of the endometrium (lining of the womb) in the second stage of the menstrual cycle.
- Help regulate menstruation.
- Change the mucus produced by the glands in the cervix so that it becomes thick and acidic, thus protecting a potential pregnancy from infection.
- Aid development of the glands in the breast.
- Increase water and salt retention, which may lead to painful breasts and weight gain.
- Improve the immune system.
- Have a relaxant effect on some of the muscles in the body (i.e. stomach, uterus, and fallopian tubes).
- Increase production of sebum, leading to more oily skin and spots.

In addition, progesterone may have an impact on mood, leading to an increased irritability. Hence, women often report experiencing changes in mood prior to having a period when the levels of progesterone are at their highest.

Testosterone and androstenedione

Both female and male sex hormones are produced by men and women, but at different levels. Up until the menopause, women have about one-tenth of the amount of male sex hormones that are found in men.

Both testosterone and androstenedione are produced in the ovary, and after the menopause, these hormones go on being produced for a few years. In addition, androstenedione is produced by the adrenal glands (on top of each kidney). The amount of androstenedione produced by the adrenal glands is unchanged after the menopause, although after the menopause it is converted to a form of oestrogen (oestrone) in the fatty tissue.

The role of male hormones in women is not fully understood, although they have been shown to:

- Increase libido.
- Stimulate the growth of pubic, facial and underarm hair.
- Possibly enhance mood.
- Increase the density of specific bones (for example, the hip bone).

As can be seen from the above lists, both male and female hormones have a number of functions within the body. Although levels of these hormones change around the time of the menopause, this does not happen suddenly. Ovarian changes occur from around the age of 35 until around the age of 55 to 60 years.

Body changes leading to the menopause

A woman is born with around seven million ovarian follicles, containing egg cells. This number decreases from birth, until there are none remaining after the menopause. The reduction in the number of follicles is more rapid once women reach their mid-thirties and by the mid-forties, there are significantly reduced numbers of follicles. Over the next few years the body increases its efforts to stimulate the remaining follicles to produce egg cells. At this time, menstruation may become irregular or may change so that it is heavier or lighter than usual.

As women enter their forties, the ovarian follicles become less sensitive to stimulation by the hormone, follicle-stimulating hormone (FSH), which is produced by the pituitary gland beneath the base of the brain. Although the pituitary gland increases the production of FSH, ovulation does not always occur during each menstrual cycle.

During the years that women approach the menopause, the production of follicle-stimulating hormone can reach 10–15 times more than that which occurs at the time of the menopause. A blood test to measure the level of follicle-stimulating hormone may be carried out to determine whether a woman is approaching the menopause. However, since the levels of this hormone can fluctuate considerably, it is usually necessary to repeat the test over a period of time to be sure that ovulation has not recommenced. Many doctors feel that the reliability of this blood test is not good enough to make it of much value in determining whether or not a woman is approaching the menopause.

Although ovulation does not necessarily occur during each cycle prior to the menopause, women continue to menstruate since the ovary produces enough oestrogen to stimulate the growth of the lining of the womb. Bleeding occurs when

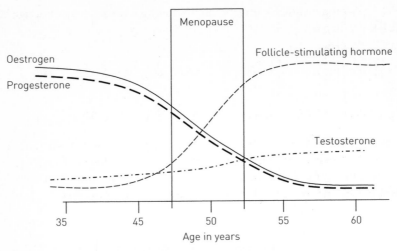

Figure 1.2. Changes in hormone levels over the years.

the oestrogen level falls. However, periods tend to be irregular, painless and heavy in cycles where ovulation does not occur.

Changes in the length of the menstrual cycle frequently occur in the time leading up to the menopause. Women sometimes notice that their cycle becomes shorter, often lasting for just 18–24 days. This is usually followed by a lengthening of the cycle duration, with occasional periods being missed. Eventually, as the menopause occurs, the periods stop altogether.

As can be seen in Figure 1.2, from around the age of 30 years, levels of oestrogen and consequently, progesterone, start to fall. Although initially there is quite a gradual decline in oestrogen production, the rate of decline speeds up around the menopause.

The term 'menopause' literally means the cessation of menstruation, and it occurs when the body has exhausted its supply of ovarian follicles containing eggs. Once the ovarian follicles cease to exist, the hormone oestrogen is no longer produced in the large quantities needed to stimulate growth of the lining of the womb (endometrium) in preparation for fertilisation. Thus, much smaller quantities of oestrogen are produced and menstruation ceases. Doctors tend to define women as menopausal once they have ceased to menstruate for 12 consecutive months.

When does the menopause occur?

The average age of the menopause in Britain is 51 years, with most women becoming menopausal between the ages of 45 and 55 years. Eighty per cent of women will have reached the menopause by the age of 54 years. A number of factors have been found to contribute to the age of menopause:

- Smoking – women who smoke tend to experience the menopause on average, $1\frac{1}{2}$ to 2 years earlier than women who do not smoke.
- Weight – women with a greater body mass tend to have a later menopause than thinner women.
- Genetics – mothers and daughters tend to experience the menopause at a similar age.

In addition to factors contributing to the age of the menopause, a very small proportion of women experience what is called, 'premature menopause', where menstruation ceases before the age of 40 years.

Premature menopause

The cause of premature menopause is largely unknown, but it occurs when the ovaries fail to respond to stimulation by the pituitary gland. The pituitary gland produces the hormones, follicle-stimulating hormone and luteinising hormone, which are necessary for the production of the ovarian hormones oestrogen and progesterone. Thus, women experiencing a premature menopause will have high blood levels of follicle-stimulating hormone and luteinising hormone, but the ovaries do not produce ovarian follicles. Without ovarian follicles, oestrogen levels fall and progesterone is not produced.

Premature menopause can occur at any age before 40 years, and may even happen shortly after menstruation begins. Although very few women (just one per cent) experience premature menopause, those who do may suffer considerable distress. In addition to experiencing symptoms such as hot flushes, night sweats and vaginal dryness, women who experience a premature menopause are often concerned about their ability to have children. Although in the past, women were advised that they would not be able to conceive, advances in fertility technology mean that it may now be possible to achieve a pregnancy. In particular, treatment with a fertilised ovum from a donor may be possible. In addition, ovarian function has been shown to recommence in a few women, either spontaneously, or while taking hormone replacement therapy. Even so, the chances of becoming pregnant remain low.

The physical effects of reduced oestrogen levels

Many areas of the body are sensitive to oestrogen and therefore a reduction in oestrogen gives rise to a number of physical changes. The areas of the body sensitive to oestrogen include:

- Breasts.
- Blood vessels and the heart.
- Bones.
- Brain.
- Urinary organs (bladder and urethra).
- Genital organs (uterus, vagina and vulva).
- Skin.
- Hair.

Breasts

Before reaching the menopause, the breast tissue changes during each menstrual cycle and often results in women experiencing tender breasts during the days before a period starts. For some women, the breasts feel lumpy, especially near the armpits. After the menopause, these cyclical changes in breast tissue stop and the breasts feel soft, less firm and not lumpy.

The risk of breast cancer increases with age, and although all women are encouraged to carry our regular breast checks to look for changes, this becomes even more important as women get older. Although many breast changes are harmless and do not require further action, it is important to have any changes investigated, as there is a small chance that it could be the first signs of cancer. Any changes in the breasts, therefore, should be reported to the doctor as a matter of urgency. If there is a cancer present, treatment is more effective if started early.

Women should be aware of how their breasts normally look and feel, so that during everyday activities such as bathing, showering and dressing, they can detect any changes at an early stage. In 1998, the Department of Health issued a paper called *Be Breast Aware*, where a five-point code of breast awareness stated that women should:

(1) Know what is normal for them.

(2) Become familiar with the look and feel of their own breasts.

(3) Know what changes to look for.

(4) Report any changes without delay.

(5) Attend three-yearly breast screening once they reach the age of 50 years.

In particular, changes that women should observe for are:

- Changes in the shape of the breast, especially when caused by arm movements or by lifting the breasts.
- Any puckering or dimpling in the skin.

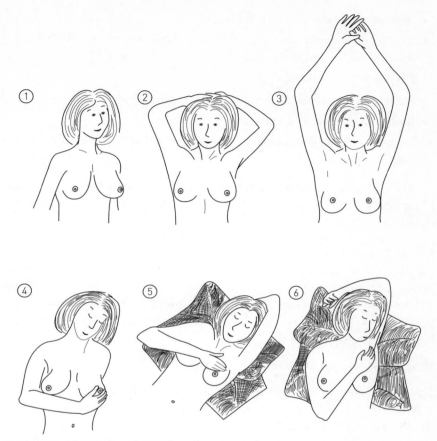

Figure 1.3. Carrying out self breast examination

Step one: Stand in front of the mirror with your hands by your sides or on your hips and look for any differences there may be between the two breasts. Then place your hands on your hips with your elbows pointing outwards and press inwards until your chest muscles tighten. Look carefully for any changes in the shape of your breasts, turning from side to side and leaning forward.

Step two: Raise your hands above your head and look for any changes in the appearance of your breasts.

Step three: Stretch your arms above your head, again looking for any changes in your breasts.

Step four: Check the nipples for any changes.

Step five: Many women find that the shower is a good place to carry out this and the next step. Some women, however, may find it easier lying down on the bed. Raise your left arm and use your fingers of your right hand to explore the left breast. Do not squeeze or prod the breast, but instead, keep your fingers together and use them flat to feel every part of the breast. Do the same with the other breast.

Step six: Again, using your fingers, feel between the breast and the armpit and then the area leading up to the collar bone.

- Any new discomfort or pain in one breast.
- Any lumps or bumpy areas in one breast or armpit, which appear different from the other breast or armpit.
- Discharge from the nipple.
- Bleeding or moist areas of the nipple that don't heal easily.
- Rashes on or around the nipple.
- Any change in nipple position, such as being pulled in, or pointing in a different direction.

Many women find it convenient to carry out self-checks of their breasts when preparing for a bath or a shower. Figure 1.3 may help to guide you through the steps of breast examination.

In addition to breast awareness, from the age of 50 years, women are advised to have a mammogram every three years. This is an X-ray procedure, which can detect any breast changes at an early stage. Because the breast tissue prior to the menopause is dense, it is difficult to accurately detect any breast changes, and therefore mammography is not routinely offered to women under the age of 50.

Blood vessels and the heart

Up until the menopause, heart disease is five times more common in men than it is in women. Following the menopause, however, there is a sharp increase in the incidence of heart disease amongst women. The mechanisms that increase women's risk of heart disease after the menopause are still not fully understood, and research is ongoing in this area. Studies suggest, however, that oestrogen affects the heart through its ability to influence the blood cholesterol level, the clotting mechanism, the blood vessel walls, and the production of insulin.

Research has shown that after the menopause, there is anything between a two and twenty per cent increase in blood cholesterol level, suggesting that oestrogen reduces the level of cholesterol in the blood. In addition, a further fat found in the blood (triglycerides) has been found to increase by between seven and thirty-five per cent after the menopause. The body's supply of oestrogen, therefore, appears to protect women against the development of atherosclerosis (where the blood vessels get 'furred up'). Furring up of the blood vessels, not only reduces the amount of blood that can get to important organs, such as the brain and the heart, but also increases the risk of a thrombosis (a blood clot) occurring in the blood vessels leading to these organs. Studies have also found that oestrogen acts directly on the blood vessel walls, causing dilation of the vessels, and therefore improving the blood supply to vital organs such as the heart and the brain.

The clotting mechanism in the body is complex, with a number of different clotting factors acting in different ways to decrease and increase clotting as the need arises. Studies have shown that before the menopause women are less likely than men to experience arterial thrombosis (blood clots), and therefore, the body's oestrogen appears to be protective against this type of blood clot.

Older women have been shown to be less able to control the breakdown of carbohydrates, and consequently the body produces higher levels of insulin. Research has suggested that not only is this reduction in control over carbohydrates linked to low levels of oestrogen, but that it is an important mechanism in the development of heart disease.

See also Chapter 5 for other factors influencing heart disease and ways of minimising the risks, and Chapter 8 for the impact of HRT on heart disease.

Bones

Bone is a living tissue, and is constantly changing in structure. In adults, the entire skeleton is completely replaced every 7 to 10 years. There are two mechanisms within the body that maintain bone formation. Firstly, the bone is formed by *osteoblast* cells, using minerals such as calcium; and secondly, the bone is resorbed by *osteoclast* cells, which maintain the shape of the growing bone. These two mechanisms are kept in balance by hormones such as oestrogen, parathyroid and calcitonin.

In both men and women, bone mass rises from childhood, until it peaks around the late twenties. Over the following ten years or so, the balance between bone formation and bone breakdown stays stable. After this, from the age of around 40, both men and women gradually start to lose bone mass as part of the general ageing process. For women, however, bone loss is more rapid and accelerates in the years after the menopause. When oestrogen levels fall around the time of the menopause, the rate of bone resorption by osteoclast cells increases, but the rate of bone formation by osteoblast cells remains the same. Hence, there is a gradual loss in bone mass. For some women, the bone mass falls significantly and the bones become thin and vulnerable to being broken. This is termed 'osteoporosis' or 'brittle bone disease'. The rate of bone loss increases in the years immediately after the menopause, with up to 20 per cent of bone loss occurring in the first 10 years after menopause. The rate of bone loss slows thereafter.

Osteoporosis generally affects the spine first, with crush fractures resulting in a loss of height, curving of the spine and long-term backache. A woman's risk of developing osteoporosis, and consequent broken bones, depends on the peak bone mass (the peak bone density that is reached in the late twenties), and the rate of bone loss. Peak bone mass is increased by factors such as a diet rich in calcium and weight-bearing exercise. The age and rate of bone loss is influenced by factors such as the menopause, family history, smoking, and excessive alcohol intake. A woman's chances of sustaining hip fracture doubles if her mother has a history of hip fracture.

See also Chapter 5 for further information about factors influencing osteoporosis and ways of reducing the chances of developing this disease.

Brain

Oestrogen has been found to be necessary for the maintenance of healthy tissue in a number of areas of the brain, in particular the area of the brain responsible for memory. This area of the brain is also the place that becomes diseased during Alzheimer's disease (see Chapter 5).

In addition to memory, a number of studies have shown that oestrogen improves mood. Progestogens, however, which are synthetic forms of progesterone, have been found to decrease some of the positive effects of oestrogen on mood. But it is important to note that low mood is very different from a clinically diagnosed depressive disorder: they arise from the alteration of different mechanisms within the brain. Indeed, studies have shown that women with clinical depression tend to get worse when taking oestrogen replacement therapy.

In much the same way that the body's oestrogen appears to be protective against heart disease, it also seems to offer some protection against strokes.

The urinary organs

The body's supply of oestrogen has been shown to influence many aspects of the urinary organs. It maintains the pliability and softness of the lining of the urethra (the tube from where urine is passed), it maintains the elasticity of the bladder, and it possibly decreases the irritability of the urethral and bladder muscle. After the menopause, therefore, women may experience problems with incontinence, frequency in passing urine and urgency in passing urine.

The genital organs

Oestrogen maintains the thickness and lubrication of the lining of the vagina and stimulates the production of useful vaginal bacteria, which help to prevent infection. In addition, oestrogen maintains the acid level in the vagina at a level where these useful vaginal bacteria can survive. After the menopause, therefore, women may experience an increase in vaginal infections. They may also experience vaginal dryness, making sexual intercourse uncomfortable or painful.

Skin and hair

Although women often report skin and hair changes when taking hormone replacement therapy, relatively few studies have been carried out to prove whether there is a link between oestrogen and the skin and hair. In addition, the few studies that have been carried out often report conflicting results. Nevertheless, the general findings are that oestrogen increases the collagen (elasticity) level in the skin and enhances the blood supply to the skin. It has also been suggested that oestrogen increases the lifespan of the hair follicle, which is presumably why women report thinning and drying of the hair after the menopause.

Summary

- The normal menstrual cycle is divided into three phases: the follicular, the luteal and the menstrual phase. During these phases varying amounts of the female hormones oestrogen and progesterone are produced.

- Women also produce the male hormones testosterone and androstenedione. The role of these hormones in women is unclear.

- Ovarian changes do not suddenly occur at the menopause, but start around the age of 35 and go on until age 55 to 60.

- In Britain, the average age of the menopause is 51 years, with most women having reached it by the age of 54 years.

- A small proportion of women will experience a premature menopause before the age of 40 years.

- Oestrogen and progesterone have many functions within the body. After the menopause, when significantly lower amounts of female hormones are produced, a number of body changes are experienced. Particular areas of the body that are sensitive to oestrogen are the breasts, blood vessels, heart, bones, brain, urinary organs, genital organs, skin and hair.

Experiencing symptoms during the menopause

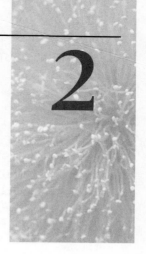

Although for some women, the only sign of the menopause is the cessation of menstruation, the majority of women report experiencing additional symptoms. In particular, women most frequently report experiencing hot flushes, night sweats, tiredness, aching joints and emotional disturbances.

While it has been suggested that there are over one hundred symptoms associated with the menopause, only hot flushes, night sweats and urogenital symptoms (for example, frequency and urgency in passing of urine, and vaginal dryness) have been shown to have a definite link with changing levels of oestrogen. This does not, however, mean that other symptoms are any less important. Nor does it mean that these symptoms are *not* related to the menopause. It simply means that a link has not been found between many of the symptoms frequently experienced during the menopause and changing oestrogen levels.

Although many menopausal symptoms are likely to be caused by a lowered oestrogen level, they also appear to be influenced by a number of social and cultural factors. For example, studies have shown that women from a lower social class report more severe symptoms than their higher social class counterparts. In addition, women experiencing a higher level of satisfaction in their relationship with a partner have been found to experience a lower level of menopausal symptoms. It is difficult to know, however, whether relationship dissatisfaction *causes* a higher level of menopausal symptoms or whether menopausal symptoms *lead to* dissatisfaction with relationships. While the main focus in this chapter is on the experience of menopausal symptoms, the impact of a number of social changes on the menopause is equally important, and therefore discussed in detail in Chapter 4.

What symptoms may I get during the menopause?

One of the first signs that women notice when approaching the menopause is a change in the pattern and heaviness of their menstrual periods. By the age of 45 years, it is common for the menstrual cycle to shorten in duration, with cycles being as short as 18 to 21 days. Following this, the cycle tends to get longer, with women often going for 2 or 3 months without a period. Some months later, menstruation stops altogether. Over this time, women may start to notice hot flushes and, in particular, they experience them at the time of menstruation, when the levels of oestrogen in the body are lowest.

The most frequently reported symptoms are:

- Hot flushes.
- Night sweats.
- Tiredness.
- Alterations in sleep patterns.
- Difficulty in concentrating.
- Poor memory.
- Emotional disturbances.
- Aches and pains in joints.
- Vaginal dryness.
- Decrease in libido.
- Urinary symptoms (frequency in passing urine and recurrent urinary infections).
- Crawling sensation under the skin.

How many women experience symptoms?

As discussed in the introductory chapter, throughout this book the results of a large survey and interview-based study (the *Women's Health Study*) will be drawn upon to illustrate women's personal experiences of the menopause.

While around three-quarters of women report experiencing some menopause-related symptoms, most do not rate these as severe. As can be seen in Figure 2.1, in the *Women's Health Study* survey, around one-fifth of women described their symptoms as being severe. The most frequently reported symptoms were hot flushes, night sweats, and tiredness. Of these symptoms, night sweats seemed to cause the most distress, with over one-third of women stating that they experienced severe night sweats.

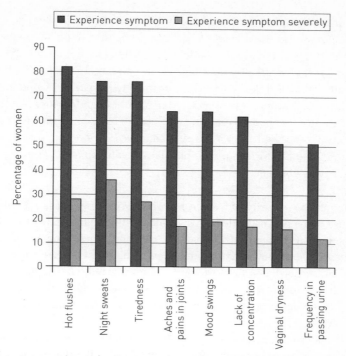

Figure 2.1. Experience and severity of symptoms experienced by 413 women aged 51–57 years, in the *Women's Health Study* survey.

How might these symptoms affect me?

Women's experiences of the menopause vary greatly, and are often influenced by social and cultural factors. Nevertheless, by using women's accounts of their experiences, gathered during the *Women's Health Study* interviews, it is possible to present an overall picture of the ways in which the menopause may be experienced.

The onset of symptoms

Although the average age of the menopause is 51 years, most women report experiencing symptoms from age 45 onwards. Symptoms, therefore, tend to occur over a number of years, often being quite subtle when they start. Since the only sure sign that women have reached the menopause is the cessation of menstruation for 12 consecutive months, recognition of symptoms as 'menopausal' may occur after the event. When looking back over the past few years, women are often able to recall experiencing slight symptoms, for which they could not identify a cause. Having then stopped menstruating, it becomes easier to recognise these previously experienced symptoms were related to the menopause:

❝I don't think that you are aware of the changes. I'm 53, coming on for 54 now ... it started when I was 45 really, to be honest. But it's little things, but at the time you don't realise what it is. Things like not being able to think properly. That was the initial thing – lack of interest in things really. It was all rather subtle at the beginning. It wasn't anything definite. And then about 2 years after, when I was 47, 48, I started having quite heavy periods. They suddenly started getting really heavy .... And I thought, that's funny, what's going on? And then I got a lot of headaches .... And quite a lot of mood swings. I'd go from being quite normal to really quite down in the dumps, which I was not used to.❞

Although the majority of women report experiencing a gradual onset of the menopause, some get very little in the way of warning signs. Rather than noticing slight changes in their menstrual pattern, therefore, these women experience a sudden onset of quite severe symptoms. In particular, hot flushes can start rather abruptly. Since hot flushes are thought to be triggered by swings in oestrogen levels, rather than a low oestrogen level *per se*, it seems likely that these women experience a sudden drop in hormone levels, making symptoms not only sudden, but also severe.

Women who have a hysterectomy, with or without the removal of ovaries, also tend to experience a sudden onset of symptoms shortly after the operation. For this reason, doctors often recommend insertion of an oestrogen implant, at the time of the operation. See Chapter 8 eight for further information about different types of hormone replacement therapy.

Changes in menstruation

Probably the most obvious sign that women associate with the menopause is a change in their normal menstrual pattern. Irregular bleeding usually occurs when women do not ovulate. Without ovulation, the ovary does not produce progesterone and therefore the lining of the womb is not shed properly at the end of the cycle. However, whilst oestrogen is still being produced, the lining of the womb will continue to grow. Having thickened, this womb lining cannot be maintained forever and, therefore, it falls away in an erratic way, causing irregular bleeding.

Thus, women, who have in the past experienced very regular menstrual cycles, may notice that they have both long and short gaps in between menstruating:

❝I might go 2 or 3 months without a period and would think ... well that's it, but no! Also they were heavier. They would last for seven days and then I would have a couple of weeks without and then I would have another one. So it always seemed as if I was having a period all the time ... almost. And then they started spreading out so that the gaps between were 2 or 3 months and I thought ... Oh this is it. Then I went a year without one. **"**

In addition to an irregular menstrual pattern, most women report an increase in the heaviness of their periods during the time leading up to the menopause:

"I started having my periods 2 or 3 days late, and they would be extremely heavy ... floods and having to really think on the first couple of days what I was going to be doing because I couldn't be that far away from a toilet. Errrm that went on for a couple of years and then when I was ... between 50 and 51, I went from the September to the January without a period. Then I had just one in November and no more after that. **"**

The definition of heavy menstrual bleeding is the loss of over 80 ml of blood in one menstrual cycle. The most likely causes of heavy bleeding in women of menopausal age are hormonal changes or possibly fibroids (balls of muscle that grow inside the uterus) (see Chapter 3). Although heavy bleeding may be a normal feature of the menopause and often does not require medical investigation, women who experience sudden heavy periods, or bleeding between cycles, should always seek medical advice. The risk of endometrial cancer (cancer of the lining of the womb) increases after the age of 40 years, and one of the first signs that a woman will notice is a change in bleeding pattern. If prompt medical attention is sought, however, endometrial cancer can usually be treated effectively.

Some women find the excessive bleeding difficult to manage and may prefer to seek treatment. A growing number of treatment options are available to women, including medication, hysterectomy or more recently, endometrial ablation or resection (removal of the lining of the womb) (see Chapter 3).

Although most women notice that their periods get heavier prior to the menopause, a few women report that they get lighter. This change in menstrual flow may then be followed by lengthening gaps between periods, until they finally cease:

"And then my periods got lighter, and that was unusual. And so I thought, hello, this [the menopause] is definitely happening now. And when I was about 50 I suppose, they started missing the odd month here and there and errm ... then, when I was 52, I had a period as normal and then I never saw another one .... That was it, finished! Very smooth. **"**

Eventually, whether spontaneously or because of surgical intervention, all women stop having periods. Although it has been suggested that the absence of periods can make women feel less feminine, most women seem to welcome not having to deal with what they see as the inconvenience of menstruation. While menstruation may be viewed as useful when it represents fertility, once this stage of a woman's life is considered complete, women are generally happy when their periods stop:

> **❝**I found that having periods was just a bind anyway. You get past the age of reproduction . . . well past the age where you want to reproduce and you just think that the whole thing is a chore after that. What's the point of it? Just turn the tap off and when somebody turned the tap off, it was wonderful.**❞**

For most women, the end of menstruation means a greater freedom. Not only are women able to live their lives without the inconvenience that menstruation can bring, but once the menopause becomes established, they also are free from the possibility of pregnancy (also see Chapter 9):

> **❝**I didn't feel that I was any less of a woman because I didn't have periods anymore. I didn't ever feel like that. It's quite liberating not having periods any more. You don't have to think about what time of the month it is or whether you can go here or there . . . and there's no risk of pregnancy anymore, so from that point of view, it's a lot better. I can't say that ever looked upon becoming post-menopausal as a problem.**❞**

While most women interviewed expressed happiness about stopping menstruation, one or two women sensed that a loss of menstruation was associated with feeling less feminine:

> **❝**And believe it or not . . . the ceasing of periods . . . although it's nice to be able to say, well I'm going swimming or whatever . . . but I do miss them as such. I don't feel as feminine. When I speak to other girls in work and I say to them 'I actually miss mine [periods]'. And they say that I must be absolutely mad. But I actually do, I miss it. I miss feeling feminine.**❞**

Hot flushes and night sweats

The most frequently reported symptoms associated with the menopause are hot flushes and night sweats, with over three-quarters of women stating that they experience these symptoms. Hot flushes occur most frequently during the year after menstruation ceases and are thought to be a result of swings in oestrogen levels. Thus, once oestrogen production has settled at the lower level found some time after the menopause, hot flushes should cease.

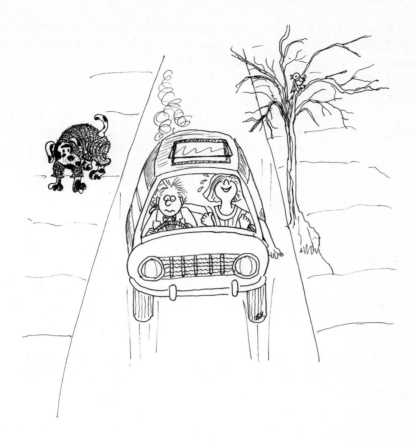

Hot flushes are associated with dilation of the blood vessels in the face, neck and hands, with an increased skin temperature in these areas. The frequency of hot flushes has been shown to increase in hot weather and to decrease in women taking regular physical exercise. A Swedish study of women aged 52 to 54 showed that women who were physically active experienced around half the amount of flushes as women who were not physically active. This may be related to an increased level of brain chemicals, called endorphins, which are released during exercise.

The length of time that women experience hot flushes can vary enormously, with some women having them for just a few months and others experiencing them for a few years. Occasionally, women continue to have hot flushes for up to ten years after they have reached the menopause. The severity of the flushes, however, tends to lessen as time goes on. In addition to variations in the duration, the intensity of flushing differs amongst women. Some women report little more than a transient sense of warmth, whilst others find that their skin reddens, they feel a sudden intense heat, and they perspire profusely. The frequency of hot flushes can also vary a lot, with some women only experiencing the occasional flush and others finding that they have more than ten in any one day. On the whole, around one-third of women rate their hot flushes as severe:

> **❝**The hot flushes suddenly started and with such a vengeance ... I was actually in a new job at the time ... and its really embarrassing to be sitting there, dripping everywhere. You don't quite believe it until it happens to you. I would have perspiration trickling down my back, my head would be hot, I couldn't take dictation because my hands were all wet.**❞**

For a few women, hot flushes occur so frequently that one follows shortly after another:

> **❝**I just started getting the terrible flushing and I didn't know what it was at that time. But I used to get it all the time. Literally, as soon as one went another was following. I would wash up and would absolutely pour with sweat. And I would have to get up at night and I was so tired as well because of not sleeping.**❞**

Some women also find the visibility of hot flushes embarrassing, particularly when they occur in the presence of work colleagues or around those who have not had similar experiences:

> **❝**It's very embarrassing when you get your hottie. Not so much around women, although the younger girls look at you and you think, 'Christ I'm having a hottie and she can see it'. And you just say 'Oh, it's going to pass in a minute' [laughs]. But I find it more embarrassing around men. Terribly embarrassing.**❞**

Such embarrassment is often created from concerns over being identified as old. Unfortunately, within the Western world the menopause and its association with ageing, has led to it being cast in a negative light.

Although around a third of women rate their experiences of hot flushes as being severe, for the majority they are fairly mild:

> **❝**When I started the menopause, I just got the hot flushes, but not to any great significance. I mean it didn't worry me or upset my life or do anything. I got night sweats and found them more uncomfortable than flushes during the day. I didn't find those uncomfortable. I just felt nicely warm actually.**❞**

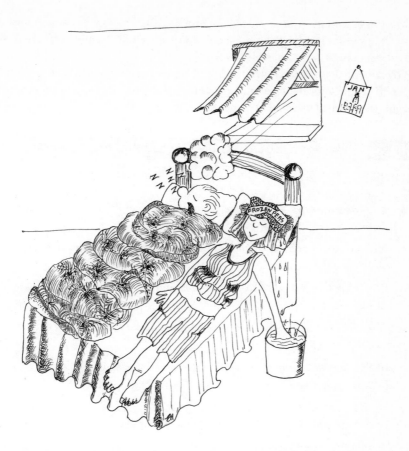

In addition to hot flushes, women frequently report experiencing night sweats, which often lead to considerable sleep disturbance:

> ❝I'd started to get the flushes. The beginnings of them wasn't so much flushes, but a peculiar sort of creeping feeling going over you as if the devil had crept over your grave. But it didn't last that long, it gradually built up into the flushes. I never changed colour, you would never know to look at me but you could feel it wash over. And the worst of all ... the thing that took me to the doctor was the night sweats. But that didn't start until after the periods had really finished. And errrm I was having to get up in the night three or four times. I would say that they were the worst part of it because they ruined the sleep obviously. You had to keep getting up and changing.❞

Since night sweats may continue for many months, and occasionally a couple of years, additional symptoms may result from an ongoing lack of sleep. As will be discussed later in the chapter, symptoms such as low mood and lack of concentration are just as likely to be caused by a lack of sleep as they are to be caused by changes in oestrogen levels.

Treatment options for hot flushes and night sweats are outlined in Box 1, although further information about hormonal replacement therapy and alternative therapies is provided in Chapters 7 and 8.

Box 1. Treatment options for hot flushes and night sweats.

Self-help

- Try to wear clothes and use bedclothes made from natural fibres such as cotton.

- Have a clean change of nightclothes by the bed so that you can change relatively easily.

- Dress in layers, so that you can remove and replace clothes easily when hot flushes occur.

- Sleep with the bedclothes loose so that you can easily turn the covers back during a flush.

- Reduce your intake of stimulants such as tea, coffee and alcohol as these may increase the frequency of hot flushes.

- Reduce your intake of sugar and cigarettes as these can cause flushes even when you are not experiencing the menopause.

- Eat plenty of fresh vegetables and soya products, as these contain plant forms of oestrogen called phyto-oestrogens (see also Chapter 7).

- When you feel a flush coming on, try to relax by taking slow deep breaths until the flush passes. Studies have shown deep breathing to be effective in reducing flushes.

Therapies

- A number of alternative therapies, such as phyto-oestrogens (the plant form of oestrogen), evening primrose oil, and black cohosh, may be useful for the relief of hot flushes and night sweats. (See Chapter 7 for full details.)

- Hormone replacement therapy has been found to be more effective in relieving hot flushes and night sweats than any other symptom.

Tiredness

Many of the women surveyed reported feeling a lot more tired than they used to. This may be for a variety of reasons. In addition to losing sleep because of night sweats, changes in oestrogen levels may also affect a woman's ability to sleep. Women may also experience a number of social changes at the time of the menopause and this can lead to anxiety, resulting in a reduced ability to sleep. Tiredness may also be a more general feature of getting older.

Whatever the cause, many women report a decreased ability to sleep and an increased tiredness at the time of the menopause:

> **"**But I do feel that I get more tired ... and at the same time I find that I don't sleep quite as well as I used to. But then again that might be due to age. I tend to get on with it more and get through the night being unsettled. I always used to be able to sleep for 8 hours straight off but I find that I don't do that now.**"**

For a few women, the tiredness can be so great that they find themselves falling asleep, even when in the company of others:

> **"**Well I found that I got really, really tired. My son used to come and visit me and be sitting here like you are now and then I'd suddenly wake up. And I'd be talking to them and I'd go to sleep. I couldn't keep my eyes open.**"**

Some women noticed that they had more dreams during the time that they were going through the menopause. Studies have also shown that even before the menopause, women report an increased number of dreams prior to menstruation. Whilst this may be due to their increased ability to recall dreams when sleeping less heavily, it does seem feasible that there might be a hormonal link, either with lighter sleep or with increased frequency of dreams.

> **"**I mean I have always been a bad sleeper, but just lately, I've had more night-time dreams. Sometimes I sleep like a log and other nights, I'm all over the place.**"**

It is also possible that symptoms such as tiredness and changes in mood may be attributable to other conditions. Around the time of the menopause, a number of women suffer from a condition called hypothyroidism, where the thyroid gland in the neck does not produce enough of the hormone, thyroxine. One of the first signs that get reported to the doctor by people suffering with hypothyroidism is an increasing tiredness. Since this is also a symptom frequently reported by women going through the menopause, diagnosis may be delayed. Hypothyroidism can, however, be diagnosed by a simple blood test which measures the amounts of thyroid hormones being produced. If the thyroxine levels are found to be low, they can be replaced by taking tablets each day.

Although treatment options for tiredness will be largely dependent upon the cause, Box 2 provides an outline of ways in which sleep can be improved.

Box 2. Treatment options for improving sleep.

Self-help

- Avoid caffeinated drinks in the evenings.

- Avoid drinking large quantities of alcohol as this may induce early wakening.

- Try having a milk drink prior to going to bed.

- Avoid stimulating activities, such as work, in the evening.

- Try to take regular exercise as this helps to release endorphins, which may aid sleep. Avoid exercising for around two hours prior to sleeping.

- People often find that listening to story tapes in bed can help when trying to get to sleep. This is particularly helpful if there are things on your mind that are preventing you from falling asleep as the story can take your mind off other thoughts.

Therapies

- Herbal remedies such as valerian are said to contain substances that have a calming and relaxing action. In addition, aromatherapy, using an oil such as lavender, may be helpful. The oil can be used by burning it in a special aromatherapy burner, or by placing a few drops of the oil on a handkerchief under your pillow.

- Hormone replacement therapy may be useful, especially when sleep is disturbed by night sweats.

- Sleeping tablets. These generally work by increasing relaxation and reducing arousal from sleep. However, studies suggest that most sleeping tablets are unable to increase the total sleep time by much more than half an hour a night. The effectiveness of sleeping tablets is generally reduced over time.

Poor memory and lack of concentration

A number of the women interviewed said that they had noticed a change in their ability to remember things. As with other symptoms, however, women suggested that it was difficult to know whether this was directly linked to the menopause, or whether it was part of getting older.

> **"**I always had a good memory and then I was like ... 'What did I do?' You know when you go to the fridge and you wonder what it was that you wanted.**"**

In addition to memory loss, poor concentration can be problematic, especially when it interferes with work:

> **"**Things like, loss of concentration ... this was one of the first things that I noticed. You know I was working in a department store ... and I suddenly found that I was not concentrating properly. I used to daydream a lot.**"**

Whilst poor concentration and memory loss may be related to falling oestrogen levels, a lack of sleep can also give rise to these symptoms. As outlined in Box 2, there are a number of ways in which sleep can be improved, and these may also help to improve memory and concentration.

Aches and pains in joints

It has been suggested that one of the first signs of the menopause is an overall aching of the joints. Although almost two-thirds of the women in the *Women's Health Study* survey reported experiencing aches and pains in their joints around the time of the menopause, these were not generally rated as being severe. Indeed, at interview, most women put their aching joints down to the usual 'creakiness' associated with getting older. In particular, women reported feeling some joint stiffness in the morning when they got out of bed, although this generally improved as the day went on. Many women took cod liver oil for their 'creaky joints', feeling that this generally helped with lubrication.

> **"**I always remember that we were made to take a spoonful of cod liver oil when we were younger ... and I used to hate it! But I did know that it sort of helped the joints a bit ... sort of like oiling them. And so when I started getting a bit creaky I thought well, I will try that. And that was about 6 or 7 years ago. I did actually feel that it helped. Whether it's in the mind or not, I don't know, but I felt that it did help slightly.**"**

While the majority of women believed that their aching joints were due to general ageing, some reported experiencing more severe painful joints, which they felt were related to the menopause:

> ❝Over the last year I have been having problems with aches and pains. I had knee problems, ankle problems . . . oh and finger problems. Before that, I didn't have any menopausal problems at all – my periods were normal, everything was fine. And then I had one [period] on the day my dad died and nothing since. But ever since then, I've been having these problems with aching joints.❞

This woman also found that her joint pains were considerably better once she had commenced a diet that was high in phyto-oestrogens (the plant form of oestrogen – see Chapter 7 for more details about phyto-oestrogens).

Emotional disturbances

One of the main difficulties in identifying emotional disturbances as 'menopausal' is that it is too easy for women to be labelled as emotionally unstable *because* of the menopause and to ignore any other possible cause for their problems. However,

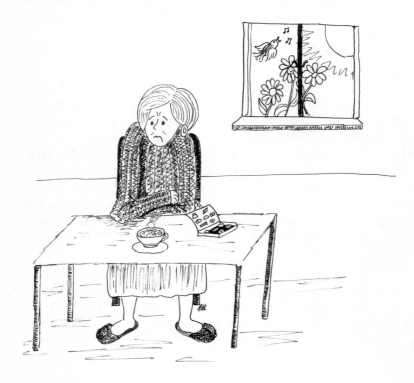

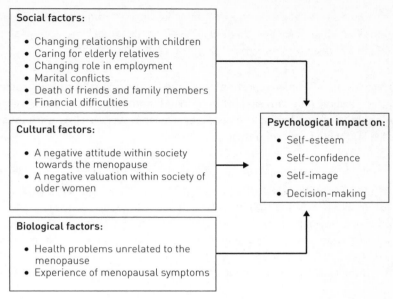

Figure 2.2. Factors influencing the psychological impact of the menopause.

many women themselves *do* view some of the emotional problems that occur at the time of the menopause as being linked to hormone changes and it would be equally inaccurate to ignore this.

Numerous studies have tried to measure the extent to which low levels of oestrogen result in emotional disturbance. Some show that changing oestrogen levels play an important part in the experience of emotional symptoms, whereas others give more importance to the impact of social changes that are often experienced at the time of the menopause. Life changes such as, problems with teenage children, the need to care for elderly relatives, relationship difficulties and changing body image, have all been shown to contribute to the experience of emotional symptoms at the time of the menopause. Figure 2.2 above illustrates the impact of possible social, cultural and biological factors on the psychological experience of the menopause.

Since there are many factors influencing a woman's emotional wellbeing at the time of the menopause, the following discussion about possible psychological disturbances should be considered alongside the issues raised in Chapter 4 where the social and cultural factors relating to the menopause are discussed.

As with all symptoms, women's experiences of emotional disturbances vary. Although many of the women interviewed said that they experienced emotional disturbances during the menopause, some women believed themselves to be 'lucky' because they had not noticed any change in their mood:

> ❝I know some people do go through some very bad emotional times. I don't think that I had mood swings though. Well, not as far as I know [laughs]. But I think I've been very lucky.❞

The majority of women reporting emotional disturbances did not view them as being catastrophic and with support from friends and family members, they were usually able to cope with their feelings. Some women described a loss of self-esteem, often leading them to question their value in life:

> ❝I think the thing that I wasn't prepared for was this feeling of, what am I good for? I couldn't do anything right, I did all sorts of stupid things. And not being able to find the right words for things ... it's so frustrating. You feel as if you are losing your grip altogether. It's a sort of falling to pieces but you are aware that you are falling to pieces. You don't have the grip that you did have.
>
> But you *do* come through it.❞

Many women reported a loss of confidence, often finding the thought of taking on their usual activities as daunting:

> ❝I tell you another thing I've also had ... I wouldn't say it was a complete lack of confidence but I've had a sort of panicky feeling – I've had a loss of confidence, where I haven't had confidence about doing things. My husband says, don't be stupid, you've done things like that before. It's silly things like having friends for dinner. All of a sudden I think, oh no, I've got to cook – I can't do it. But other times you won't think anything of it.❞

Indeed, the combination of feeling 'panicky' and having a loss of confidence was something that many women described:

> ❝Oh I had very bad anxiousness – kind of panicky. I lost my confidence and my ability to think for myself. I would just back off from things. And I'm not like that, I'm a fighter. But it was getting so bad that anything would start me off. Any confrontation with anything, I just backed off.❞

Although all of these women experienced some change in their emotional wellbeing, which they attributed to the menopause, they generally felt that with support from others, they could manage to deal with their feelings. For a very small proportion of women, however, the changing hormone levels associated with the menopause appear to result in a significant level of depression. The following woman describes how her world completely changed when she started to go through the menopause:

> **❝**I started getting these panicking attacks. It was ridiculous ... it's very difficult to explain because it sounds silly [laughs] but you know, at work you'll suddenly be doing something and you'll then think, 'I can't do this'. It's a fear that comes over you .... It's ermm really odd really. It's not pleasant. But I felt that people didn't understand .... Well I didn't! I mean you can't expect people to understand what you're going through. It's not something that you publicly go about saying ... that you're going through the menopause. It's something that you like to keep quite private really ... well I do.
>
> But I don't know really, if I'll ever be quite the same person again, to be honest. I'm a different person to the one I was, quite a different person. If I thought that I'd go back to the person that I was when I come out the other side, then I would be quite happy. Before the menopause I was happy-go-lucky, confident and outgoing and everything seemed to be normal ... nothing sensational but it was reasonably happy. I enjoyed the family, I've got a little grandson and he's lovely and I enjoy watching him grow up .... But you know, it's just difficult now. I think that it is very apt to call it 'the change of life'. Well, it spoils your life in a way ... in a nutshell.**❞**

Although this woman has clearly experienced a lot of emotional problems while she has been going through the menopause, it is important to remember that this does not happen to the majority of women. While two-thirds of women in the *Women's Health Study* survey indicated that they experienced mood swings around the time of the menopause, only one-fifth of these women rated them as being severe. In addition, most of the women interviewed did not describe their emotional symptoms as being severe.

Many women will feel that they are able to cope with the emotional symptoms experienced at the time of the menopause and, with help from a good network of supportive, caring family members and friends, treatment is often not necessary. Since emotional problems may be influenced by troublesome menopausal symptoms or by life changes, help with dealing with these problems may prove to be effective in relieving emotional distress. For some women, therefore, treatment with hormone replacement therapy may be effective in reducing emotional symptoms. However, although oestrogen has been shown to improve mood, it is important to recognise that low mood is very different from a clinically diagnosed depressive disorder, with each occurring from alteration of different mechanisms within the brain. Indeed, studies have shown that women with clinical depression tend to get worse when taking HRT.

Box 3 outlines some of the possible treatment options that might be helpful for emotional symptoms.

Box 3. Treatment options for emotional symptoms.

Anxiety

- There are many books and tapes which may be helpful for learning relaxation techniques.

- A variety of herbal remedies are available from high-street chemists and may help reduce anxiety. For example, valerian, kava kava, and St John's wort.

Low mood

- Try to find relief for any physical symptoms such as night sweats as this is likely to improve general wellbeing.

- Regular physical exercise can help to improve mood. Exercising increases the release of brain chemicals, called endorphins, which have been found to enhance mood.

- Counselling or support groups can often be helpful as they provide an opportunity to talk through problems and find solutions to psychological difficulties.

- Problem-solving or self-help groups can provide a useful source of information and advice about the menopause. Having a better understanding about the menopause has been found to reduce emotional symptoms.

- Hormone replacement therapy, particularly in high doses, has been shown to be effective in the treatment of psychological problems in some women. However, unless emotional problems are related to a reduction in oestrogen levels, HRT may make the situation worse.

- Drugs such as antidepressants and tranquillisers may be helpful for some women. This should be discussed with your doctor.

Vaginal dryness and loss of libido

A number of studies, including the *Women's Health Study*, reveal that around one-third to a half of women report experiencing sexual problems during and after the menopause. This seems to be due to a number of factors, related both to social and to biological changes. After the menopause, a low level of oestrogen can cause the lining of the vagina to become thin and dry. Although this does not happen to all women, it leads to painful sexual intercourse, sometimes resulting in small amounts of bleeding afterwards. The presence of bothersome menopausal symptoms, including tiredness and night sweats can also have an impact on sexual desire. In addition to changes arising from a reduced level of oestrogen, life stresses such as those associated with relationship or work difficulties may also reduce the desire for a sexual relationship.

Although some of the women interviewed spoke about experiencing vaginal dryness, the key concern was a lack of sexual desire, with almost half of the women interviewed experiencing a drop in libido:

> **"**I've really gone off sex in a big way and we have put that down to . . . well it must be sort of menopause. I mean, I will suffer it but I don't enjoy it and I'm just hoping that that's something that doesn't go on . . . . Very occasionally, you do think you want it [sex] and enjoy it, but quite honestly, most of the time I can take it or leave it. That's terrible, but it's not that you don't love your partner but it's just that you don't fancy the physical act of it.**"**

While a reduced libido did not create problems for all women, it was a source of anxiety for those who had a previously active sexual relationship. Women may feel guilty about their lack of sexual interest and the impact that it has on their relationship with their husband or partner:

> **"**I mean my sex life has now altered . . . . I suppose about four years ago it [sex life] started dwindling and its got less and less. And my husband and I have always had quite good relationship, I mean it [sex] dwindles a bit as you get older . . . . That's quite normal. But the trouble is, you don't get the desire for it [sex]. And I found that very hard to come to terms with because it's made me feel that I'm not the woman that I was. And that's very soul-destroying in a way and it creates problems between my husband and me. My husband is very supportive but you know, there's a limit to what men will put up with.**"**

For some women, therefore, a fall in libido and vaginal dryness can create problems, not only in terms of the physical pain that may result, but also because of the impact that symptoms might have on relationships. Box 4 outlines possible treatment options for women experiencing sexual difficulties.

> ### Box 4. Treatment options for vaginal dryness and a decrease in libido.
>
> **Vaginal dryness**
>
> - Lubricating jelly can be purchased from the chemist, and may be helpful for relieving vaginal dryness.
>
> - Oestrogen cream, applied directly to the vagina, can be very effective in relieving vaginal dryness. Minimal amounts of oestrogen are absorbed into the bloodstream, often making this an ideal treatment for women who have concerns about taking HRT (see also Chapter 8 for information on oestrogen creams).
>
> **Decrease in libido**
>
> - Testosterone implants have been shown to be effective in increasing libido.
>
> - Hormone replacement therapy may improve libido. However, a new synthetic product called tibolone (Livial™) has been found to be particularly effective for enhancing libido as it has androgenic as well as oestrogenic and progestogenic properties.
>
> (See also, Chapter 8 for more information about hormonal products and their impact on libido.)

Urinary symptoms

As with the lining of the vagina, a decrease in oestrogen causes the lining of the urethra and the bladder to become thin. In addition, a low level of oestrogen results in a slackening of the ligaments holding up the uterus, pelvic floor and bladder. This may result in a prolapse of the internal genital organs.

Studies have shown that, following the menopause, over a quarter of women experience some form of urinary symptoms. The most frequently reported symptoms are urgency and frequency in passing urine, incontinence, and pain on passing urine. In addition, urinary infections are more common following the menopause. The *Women's Health Study* survey revealed that just over half of women reported experiencing an increased frequency in passing urine.

As with vaginal dryness, oestrogen (oestriol) cream applied to the vagina has been shown to be effective in reducing the incidence of urinary tract infections. However, the evidence to support the use of oestrogen to treat urinary frequency

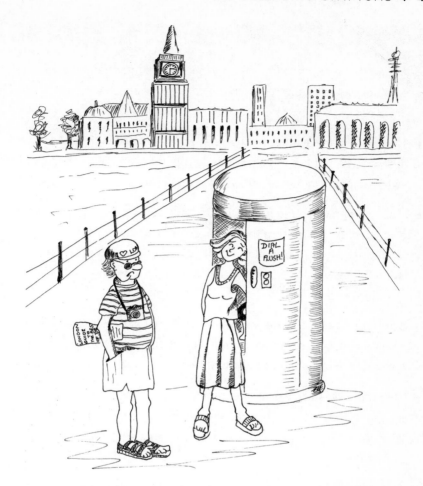

and urgency is less clear. Studies are currently investigating the role of oestrogen in these symptoms.

Crawling sensation under the skin

Although women of all ages often report skin sensations related to menstruation, this appears to be increased during the menopause. In particular, itchiness and a crawling feeling under the skin can be experienced:

> **❝**I remember having a creeping feeling up my skin. But I've not actually heard other women suffering with this. **❞**

It would seem that these skin sensations are likely to be caused by hormonal changes, although there appears to be little research into this area.

Summary

- Although the majority of women experience some menopausal symptoms, the extent to which they are experienced varies a great deal.

- There are many symptoms that may be associated with the menopause, but the most frequently reported are hot flushes, night sweats, aching joints, tiredness, and emotional disturbances.

- Most women welcome not having to have periods any longer, feeling a sense of freedom from the inconvenience of menstruation and no longer needing to worry about contraception. A small proportion of women, however, feel that the absence of periods makes them feel less feminine.

- Symptoms can interfere with work and home activities, especially when night sweats and emotional disturbances result in a lack of sleep over a prolonged period of time.

- Within the Western world, the menopause and its association with ageing is often viewed in a negative light. This can contribute to women feeling embarrassed when symptoms such as hot flushes are visible.

- A number of social, cultural and biological factors have an impact on a woman's psychological wellbeing at the time of the menopause.

- There are many ways to relieve menopausal symptoms. For some women, a change in lifestyle and diet can offer adequate symptom relief. For others, however, relief can be obtained from non-hormonal or hormonal therapies.

Treatments for heavy bleeding

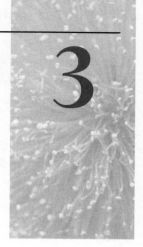

Prior to the menopause, many women experience an increased heaviness in menstruation. This may be due to hormonal changes or possibly due to fibroids. This chapter describes what fibroids are and considers both the medical and surgical treatments for heavy bleeding.

What are fibroids?

Fibroids are benign (non-cancerous) growths, which are most commonly formed in the muscle layer of the uterus. They are believed to be oestrogen-dependent (they need oestrogen to grow), because they only occur after puberty and they become smaller after the menopause. They are fairly common, with almost a quarter of women over the age of 35 having fibroids. It is not uncommon for a woman to develop more than one fibroid, and they can result in significant enlargement of the uterus.

The doctor may be able to diagnose fibroids by carrying out a pelvic examination, but often an ultrasound scan, or sometimes surgery, is needed to be sure of the diagnosis.

Many women do not experience symptoms with fibroids, often being unaware that they have them. However, they can sometimes cause heavy bleeding, which may be debilitating and lead to anaemia. If the fibroids are very large, they can cause compression of nearby organs such as the bladder or the bowel, leading to frequency in passing urine, constipation and bloating. Some women also find that particularly large fibroids cause back pain.

As can be seen in Figure 3.1, fibroids grow in different positions within the muscular wall of the uterus. They may be found in the wall of the muscle itself, or under the external lining of the wall, or they can bulge into the cavity of the uterus. The most common type of fibroid develops wholly within the muscle layer of the womb, and is called an intramural fibroid. This type of fibroid increases overall blood flow to the uterus and if large will stretch the uterus so that it increases in size. This increase in the size of the uterus typically leads to heavy bleeding.

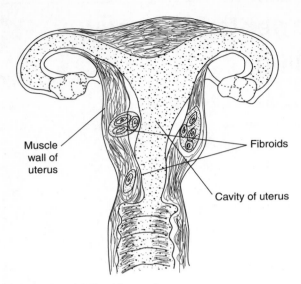

Muscle wall of uterus

Fibroids

Cavity of uterus

Figure 3.1. Typical areas of fibroid growth.

Subserous fibroids are those that project out from the outer surface of the uterus. They can grow quite large, but do not generally affect the size of the womb cavity. They are unlikely to create problems with heavy bleeding but may cause pressure on nearby organs such as the bladder and the bowel. Submucous fibroids protrude into the womb, altering its shape and sometimes filling it. As submucous fibroids grow larger, they may be expelled out of the uterus through the cervix, and become a fibroid polyp. When this happens, women often report cramp-like pains and irregular bleeding.

The majority of women with fibroids do not require treatment. In particular, women approaching the menopause may feel that they can manage the symptoms, as the fibroids will shrink after the menopause. Where fibroids cause pain, or heavy or irregular bleeding, however, women may wish to consider treatment options.

One treatment option is with specific hormone drugs that bring about an artificial menopause. This treatment works by shrinking the fibroids. Although treatment is usually effective, it can only be used on a short-term basis, and when the therapy is discontinued, the fibroid will almost always grow back. A number of unpleasant side effects may also be experienced with these drugs.

Treatment is therefore usually surgical, either by removing the uterus (hysterectomy) or the lining of the uterus (endometrial resection/ablation), or by removal of the muscle layer of the uterus (myomectomy). Recent developments have made it possible to offer women a non-surgical procedure, whereby the blood supply to the fibroid is occluded. This procedure (uterine artery embolisation) is carried out under X-ray control, and involves the insertion of a catheter into the artery supplying the fibroids and injecting a substance that stops the blood being able to reach the fibroid. The fibroid will then shrink over the following six to nine months.

Although no further treatment for fibroids is required following a hysterectomy, unfortunately, up to a third of patients having a myomectomy will require further treatment for recurrence of fibroids. The effectiveness of endometrial ablation/resection is discussed later in this chapter.

Drug therapy options for heavy bleeding

Although over half of all the hysterectomies carried out in Britain are done because of heavy bleeding, certain drug treatments have also been found to be very effective in reducing blood loss.

- Tranexamic acid. This drug works by interfering with the clotting mechanism of the blood. It has been found to be very effective in reducing menstrual bleeding and is generally tried before opting for a surgical treatment. Tablets are taken 8-hourly during menstruation. Tranexamic acid should not be used by women who have a history of deep vein thrombosis.

- Mefenamic acid. This is also a drug that interferes with the clotting mechanism by reducing the production of prostaglandin. These types of drugs are also called 'non-steroidal anti-inflammatory' drugs and have a variety of other actions, including pain relief. In addition to mefenamic acid (Ponstan), similar drugs such as indomethacin, diclofenac and ibuprofen, may also be effective in reducing blood loss. Women with a history of stomach ulcers may not be able to take these drugs and should consult their doctor for further advice.

- The combined oral contraceptive pill. The use of both progestogens and oestrogen will result in the lining of the womb (endometrium) being kept relatively thin and underactive. Thus, when this is shed during menstruation, blood loss is minimised.

- Progestogens. As discussed in Chapter 1, prior to the menopause ovulation does not occur during every monthly cycle. Without ovulation, the body does not produce progesterone, and this often leads to irregular and heavy bleeding. Progestogens can be given, therefore, over the latter half of the cycle and, when they are stopped, menstruation begins. This not only regulates menstruation, but also tends to produce a lighter period. A particularly effective way of taking progestogens, in the form of Levonorgestrel, is via an intrauterine coil. Once the coil (called a Mirena coil)

is inserted into the uterus, it releases a continuous low dose of Levonorgestrel for approximately five years. After around three months of use, the majority of women find a significant reduction in menstrual flow, often ceasing to menstruate completely. An added advantage of taking progestogens via an intrauterine device is that it also provides contraception.

In addition to medication to reduce heaviness of bleeding, iron tablets may be necessary for the treatment of anaemia.

Surgical treatment options for heavy bleeding

The two main surgical procedures for treating heavy blood loss are hysterectomy and endometrial resection or ablation. Each of these will be discussed in turn.

Hysterectomy

A hysterectomy is an operation to remove the uterus (womb). Although heavy bleeding is a key reason for women to have a hysterectomy, there are a number of other reasons. These include:

- Endometriosis, where endometrial tissue from the lining of the womb grows outside of the womb and causes pain.
- Fibroids – benign growths in the womb – which may cause heavy or painful periods.
- Cancer of the womb, cervix or ovaries.
- Ovarian cysts.
- Prolapse of the womb or bladder, where the ligaments supporting the womb or bladder become overstretched

There are three types of hysterectomy:

- A sub-total hysterectomy, where only the womb is removed and the cervix and ovaries are left in place.
- A total hysterectomy, where the womb and cervix are removed, but the ovaries are left in place.
- A total hysterectomy plus removal of ovaries and fallopian tubes.

These three types of hysterectomy are discussed in more detail below.

Sub-total hysterectomy

This is where the body of the uterus is removed, but the cervix (neck of womb) is left behind. The advantages of keeping the cervix are:

(1) The ligaments that are attached to the cervix provide some support for the vagina, and therefore the risk of a prolapse, where the vagina descends outside of the vulva is reduced. The risk of vaginal prolapse following a hysterectomy, however, is fairly low.

(2) It has been suggested that movement of the cervix during sexual intercourse results in greater sexual pleasure for women. This, however, is difficult to prove or disprove, as there are many other contributory factors to sexual enjoyment.

The disadvantages of leaving the cervix behind are:

(1) The risk of abnormal cervical smears and cervical cancer remains.

(2) Women often experience vaginal discharge from the cervix following a sub-total hysterectomy.

(3) If any endometrial tissue is left attached to the cervix, women continue to have light periods.

The cervix is rarely retained where there is evidence of malignancy (cancer).

Total hysterectomy

As already mentioned, a total hysterectomy involves the removal of the uterus and the cervix, but not the ovaries. The two main reasons for not removing the ovaries are:

(1) The woman does not wish to have her ovaries removed.

(2) The woman has not started the menopause and therefore the ovaries are still providing a good source of hormones.

Although it is unclear why, women who have a hysterectomy tend to have an earlier menopause, even though they retain their ovaries. It has been suggested that the ovaries do not function as well when there is no uterus to provide oestrogen for. It is also possible, however, that women who have a hysterectomy do so because they are experiencing heavy bleeding, and that this may be an indication of an early menopause.

Total hysterectomy plus removal of ovaries and fallopian tubes

A total hysterectomy with removal of the ovaries and fallopian tubes is largely carried out because:

(1) There is evidence of cancer.

(2) To avoid the risk of ovarian cancer.

In Britain, 5000 women per year are diagnosed as having cancer of the ovaries. Whilst this is not as high as other types of cancer, such as breast cancer, it is the seventh most commonly diagnosed cancer in women. In particular, there is a higher incidence of ovarian cancer in women over the age of 45 years. Cancer of the ovaries also tends to go unrecognised until it is at an advanced stage and therefore, doctors often advise menopausal women who are having a hysterectomy, to have their ovaries removed.

What does a hysterectomy involve?

Three different surgical techniques can be used to carry out a hysterectomy:

(1) 'Open surgery', where a cut is made into the abdomen, in order to remove the uterus.

(2) Vaginal surgery, where the uterus is removed through the vagina.

(3) Keyhole surgery, where three or four very small cuts are made into the abdomen, in order to release the uterus from its attachments, so that it can be removed through the vagina.

It may be advantageous to have a hysterectomy done using keyhole surgery, since this usually results in a shorter stay in hospital (usually around 2 or 3 days) and generally women experience less discomfort after surgery. This makes recovery quicker, with women often feeling able to return to normal activities within two weeks. However, as with any surgery, women having a keyhole hysterectomy often remain fairly tired for some 6 weeks or so.

The type of surgical technique that is most suitable will be dependent upon a number of factors. For example, if the uterus is large, it may not be possible to remove it through the vagina. In addition, a large uterus may restrict access to the blood vessels and make keyhole surgery difficult to achieve. Women who have had previous abdominal or vaginal surgery may not be able to have keyhole or vaginal surgery. If a hysterectomy is being carried out because of cancer of the uterus or ovary, an open surgical approach, where the uterus is removed through the abdomen is almost always used.

Recovering from a hysterectomy?

Immediately after the operation

The treatment following a hysterectomy will vary according to the type of surgery carried out and the reasons for the operation. A urinary catheter may be used to prevent the pressure of a full bladder from putting a strain on the surgical site. A drip, in the arm or hand may be used to provide fluids for a day or two during recovery from the operation. After an abdominal hysterectomy, a plastic tube, draining any oozing blood away from the surgical site may also be inserted.

The length of stay in hospital will also vary according to the type of operation and the speed with which recovery takes place. Generally, following an abdominal operation women need to stay in hospital for 5–8 days. If the operation is carried out vaginally or following keyhole surgery, hospital stay is usually 2 or 3 days.

Carrying out normal activities

Following discharge from hospital, the after-effects of the anaesthetic and surgery tend to make women feel tired for a few weeks. Doctors generally advise that driving be avoided for about 6 weeks following the operation, or at least until you feel able to undertake an emergency stop.

Sexual intercourse should probably be avoided for 6 weeks, giving the abdominal muscles and tissues time to heal properly.

Return to work is usual about eight weeks after the operation, although this will vary according to the type of work that is done. For example, women doing jobs that require a lot of heavy lifting may require longer away from work.

Most women feel completely well within six months.

Emotional feelings

One of the key concerns that women appear to have about a hysterectomy surrounds the possibility that the operation will leave them with a sense of feeling less of a woman. It is difficult to know where this view originates from, since the majority of women report positive experiences following a hysterectomy. In the *Women's Health Study* survey, a total of 21 per cent of women had a hysterectomy, and two-thirds of these women stated that they felt a lot better after the operation. In addition, 17 per cent of women stated that they felt a little better and 14 per cent stated that they felt the same after the operation. Just 3 per cent of women stated that they felt worse after having a hysterectomy.

During the *Women's Health Study* interviews, women who had had a hysterectomy were asked to describe how they felt after the operation. Most women said that prior to having the operation, from what they had heard, they thought that they might feel less of a woman as a result of the operation:

❝I didn't feel any different after it [hysterectomy]. And I had heard people talk about it [hysterectomy] and I had read about it and that. But I couldn't understand why they said it changed the way you felt about yourself. Because I certainly didn't feel any less of a woman. I was delighted with myself.**❞**

Some women were also concerned that having a hysterectomy might change their relationship with their husband:

> **❝**Some people said to me that you turn against your husband when you have a hysterectomy . . . and I think this was what was holding me back in the beginning . . . . My sister said that she thought I was frightened that I was not going to be a complete woman – I think she was probably right. But in the end I just had to have it [hysterectomy] done. But I think that this was what was worrying me – that there was going to be something missing. I mean, there is a lot missing (laughs). But it never caused a problem between me and my husband, never. As I said, I had it done when I was only 37.**❞**

Although there was some concern about feeling less feminine after a hysterectomy, all of the women interviewed said that this fear was unfounded:

> **❝**But it didn't worry me that I'd had the hysterectomy, and I've never regretted having it. I just thought, oh good, get shot of that, I haven't got to worry about that any longer. And my husband and I didn't have to worry about contraceptives at all. Which is lovely really.**❞**

Although women who have a hysterectomy appear to have a positive outlook on the operation, for a variety of reasons many women with heavy bleeding would rather not have a hysterectomy. Surgical developments over the past ten years or so have now made it possible for many women to avoid a hysterectomy and have just the lining of the womb destroyed (endometrial ablation or resection).

Endometrial ablation or resection

As discussed in Chapter 1, in response to ovarian hormones, the lining of the uterus, the endometrium, becomes thickened in readiness for implantation of a fertilised egg. In the absence of conception, however, the endometrium breaks down and is passed during menstruation. Destruction of the endometrium, therefore, will either significantly reduce, or eliminate menstrual bleeding.

Endometrial ablation or resection is usually carried out under hysteroscopic control, where a narrow telescope (hysteroscope) is inserted into the uterus via the vagina. Once the hysteroscope is in the uterus, the doctor is able to see the endometrium and destroy it. The operation is usually carried out under general anaesthetic, although with improvements in technique, it can be performed under local anaesthetic, with a light sedation. The procedure is often carried out in the day ward of a hospital, with most women being discharged home a few hours after having the operation.

The endometrium may be destroyed or removed, using a number of different techniques:

- Laser ablation – after distending the uterus by filling it up with fluid, laser energy is used to destroy the endometrium.

- Electrodiathermy – the endometrium is either destroyed when a rollerball electrode is passed over it, or resected when a diathermy wire loop is used to remove endometrial tissue.

- Radio frequency – radio-frequency waves are used to generate an electric field, which is then used to destroy the endometrium.

Most women are able to go home a few hours after having an endometrial ablation or resection. Some slight cramping pain is usual, for which pain-relieving drugs such as Ponstan or Paracetamol can be helpful. It is also usual to have light blood loss for a few days following the procedure and a further watery discharge for a week or two after that. If the vaginal discharge becomes coloured or offensive smelling, or low abdominal pain is experienced days after the operation, the doctor should be consulted as this may indicate that an infection has developed.

Although endometrial ablation and resection is largely effective, with around three-quarters of women reporting a significant reduction in menstrual loss, some women need the procedure repeating and, even then, may go on to have a hysterectomy. Although the procedure aims to destroy the endometrium, any tissue left behind can regenerate and cause bleeding. Because it is not possible to be sure that all of the endometrial tissue is removed, when taking hormone replacement therapy, women need to take progestogens in addition to oestrogen. This is because any remaining endometrial tissue may become cancerous if stimulated by oestrogen without protection from progestogens. See also Chapter 8 for further discussion about the risk of endometrial cancer (cancer of the lining of the womb) when taking hormone replacement therapy.

Summary

- Fibroids are non-cancerous growths generally formed in the muscle layer of the womb. Although they are fairly common in women over the age of 35, they often do not require treatment. Problematic fibroids are generally treated using surgical and X-ray image techniques.

- Heavy bleeding can be treated using drug therapies or surgical procedures.

- There are three types of hysterectomy: sub-total, total, and total plus removal of ovaries.

- There are three different surgical techniques used to carry out a hysterectomy: open abdominal, vaginal, and keyhole. The type of hysterectomy and the technique used to perform the operation will largely depend upon the reason for having the surgery.

- Most women feel well enough to leave hospital within 8 days of having a hysterectomy. Hospital stay may be reduced significantly if keyhole surgery is used.

- Most women report little emotional disturbance following a hysterectomy, often being relieved that their heavy bleeding has been resolved.

The 'change of life'

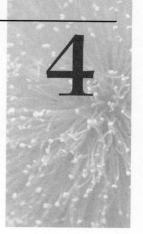

In addition to the biological changes that result from a reduction in oestrogen levels, there are a number of life changes that frequently occur around the time of the menopause. It can be difficult, therefore, to know whether menopausal symptoms are truly related to the menopause, or whether they are triggered (or made worse) by social events that coincide with the menopause.

In trying to disentangle these two aspects it has been suggested that the term 'change of life' be used to refer to all the changes (both biological and social) that occur during the middle years and that the term 'menopause' be used to describe the biological changes. There are obviously many possible social changes that may occur during the change of life, but some key changes that are reported by women are:

- Becoming a carer for elderly relatives.
- Changes in employment and finance.
- Changing relationship with children.
- Death of family or friends.
- Changes in relationships.
- Changes in body image.
- A change in outlook on life.

While the physical and life changes are not necessarily related, they may have an effect on each other. Thus, a woman might be less able to cope with symptoms such as night sweats, which often impair sleep, when she also has to deal with travelling long distances to support elderly relatives. Likewise, an ageing appearance may be more difficult to come to terms with when the loss of friends and family members serve as reminders of a woman's own mortality. Drawing on the accounts that women gave at interview, the potential impact of each of these life changes will be discussed in turn.

Caring for elderly relatives

Changes in transportation and employment over the last century have resulted in a more mobile society, with family members often living considerable distances apart. However, with an increased life expectancy, the elderly are much more likely to find themselves in need of support from their families, especially where illness has left them less able to fend for themselves.

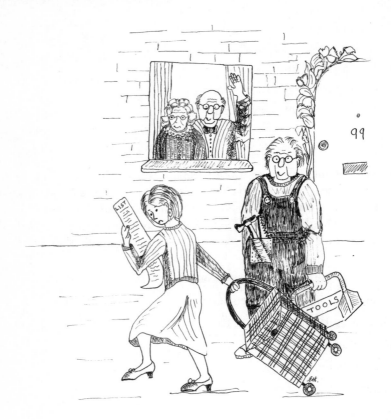

Since women usually remain the main carers for elderly relatives, whether they are biologically related or related through marriage or partnership, the impact of a mobile society is generally greater for women than for men. This increasing need for women's support, however, often arises amidst a number of other life changes. Thus, women may find themselves torn between meeting the changing demands from teenage children, or increased hours in employment, and helping to meet the needs of elderly relatives. Indeed, the need to provide some form of support for elderly relatives was frequently discussed by those women interviewed.

❝I suppose, one area of stress has been coping with my mother over the last 2 or 3 years. Coping with her living the other side of London. Her ringing up and saying things like, 'I can't turn the tap off', or something like, 'There's something wrong with my gas stove.' And knowing that you are 70 miles away and you can't do anything. I was working and trying to balance that as well as looking after my mother, it was very stressful. Feeling guilty that you were under-performing in both areas really, not doing everything that you should, either at work or at home.**❞**

Once children have left home, women can become accustomed to having more time for themselves, only to find that this extra time is then taken up by providing much-needed support for elderly relatives:

❝The kids have left home and you think, 'Oh it should all be hunky-dory now'. But we are actually caught between the children getting older and our mothers sort of becoming more dependent ... and so you kind of take on a different role, don't you?**❞**

The stress of having to deal with a number of competing time demands may result in women becoming physically ill themselves:

❝But these last few years were awful. I mean I ended up at a chiropractor ... all to do with my back. But it was tension, stress, just everything. From the business of my life at that time. My father died 5 years ago and my mother lived in Norfolk. Errrm we were up and down to Norfolk sort of looking after or keeping an eye on her. And then my mother-in-law died 3 years ago. She lived in Nottingham and so every week we were either going to Nottingham or to Norfolk. Errm and the boys [sons] were coming with us half of the time and not coming the others. But the pressure of that was hard, because they weren't really old enough to be left by themselves ... and we had gone and left them. It was stressful as you can imagine. I think I felt so grotty, so completely at the end of my tether really. It was a completely general air of errrmm hopelessness.**❞**

Having provided much support for their children over the years, women often look forward to being able to pursue their own interests more, once the children have become old enough to look after themselves. However, as the women interviewed expressed, this new-found freedom may soon be snatched away as elderly relatives require more support. Whilst women may be willing carers for elderly relatives, they also have needs of their own, often needing time to follow personal ambitions or desires. As will be seen later in this chapter, women frequently re-evaluate their life during the middle years, and this may involve fulfilling a lifelong ambition.

Changes in employment and finance

Although gender differences associated with employment exist throughout the working life, some are specific to the middle years. The cost of sending children to university is frequently cited as a reason for women to increase their hours of paid employment. For many women, this creates an extra burden as they also continue to have key responsibility for maintaining the home. However, women may have both positive and negative experiences concerning paid work. Having spent time at home bringing up children, women may view paid work as a new challenge. It often provides an opportunity to pursue a career, and may increase self-esteem or independence:

> ❝When the boys were semi-grown-up, I was out working full-time and I was becoming more independent. And I was becoming me. I had become me again instead of just being a mum . . . by going back to work full-time and having my own money – finances not being so hard . . . it alleviated a lot of the problems. But then, I think things started to fall apart, as there were crises in the family – deaths and family problems make it all difficult again.❞

Although work can offer women new opportunities, increasing the number of hours spent in paid employment may create added stress, especially as women are still expected, or feel the need, to continue having primary responsibility for looking after the family and home.

The other major employment change that women often face during midlife is early retirement. This may be taken voluntarily to meet increasing demands with elderly relatives or may occur because of redundancy. Making adjustments to retirement can, however, sometimes be difficult:

> ❝I think that stopping working was the most profound thing that changed my perception of myself. It took a long while to adjust really. And certainly it had a big impact on my level of confidence – self-confidence, that kind of thing. And trying to find a role for yourself really. In the end I sorted it out by doing a lot of voluntary work instead and that helped the transition really. And now I am perfectly content, but that was the big change that I felt.❞

The sense of not being needed any more in a work environment may be made worse when it happens at a time when children leave home and women may feel that they have less of a role to play as a mother:

❝Well it's interesting because the job that I'm in at the moment will probably fold up next year. And I think that will be quite a transition for me even at the age I am, because I've worked all my life. And I think that it is the getting up in the morning, having a shower, putting on your nice smart blouse and skirt and bombing off to work, albeit you know, a fairly modest little job. To think that errr I shan't be doing that because I'm not needed, that has a big effect on me. Because I've got so used to . . . not just being financially independent but getting away from the house and get out and use the old grey matter and be useful. I do enjoy it. This word retirement has all the connotations of old age and slippers and pipes and taking dogs for a walk and that's all you've got in life.**❞**

While both men and women may experience changes in self-image associated with retirement, for women, this occurs amidst a variety of other changes, both social and biological.

Changing relationships with children

Relationships between parents and children change as children make the transition from school to further education or employment, and move away from the parental home. This transition, however, may not be problem-free, for parents have less control over their children's actions. In addition, children who are taking examinations, or those having relationship difficulties often require emotional support:

❝Well the stress is nearly always to do with children . . . well, my daughter left her husband and came to live with us. And again this was a stressful time.**❞**

When children leave home, women experience a mixture of emotions. Some are thankful for their increasing independence, giving the parents more time to spend together:

❝Because there are some good things, you know the fact that the children are growing up. We actually are now able to go on holiday . . . on our own . . . and have been, once or twice.**❞**

Others find it quite difficult to deal with the changes brought by their children leaving home:

❝Oh I hated it when my children left home. My daughter moved out when she was 22 . . . alright she was buying her own place and she's only down the

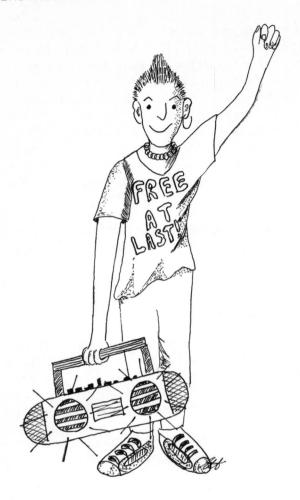

road ... but I think the crunch was that she took her bed with her and I went up into her room after she had gone and there was this empty void. I used to go and look in the room and I would burst into tears. I really did. It was like a big void. My husband couldn't understand it. I found that it took 2 or 3 weeks to get used to the idea. There wasn't all the washing and all the mess and the cooking and there wasn't all the friends coming in and out ... I think that was a lot to do with it because they used to bring friends home and all of a sudden all of that stopped and it was all quiet. It was very hard.**"**

Although many women mention missing their children once they have left home, they generally adjust to the situation fairly quickly, often finding that there are advantages as well as disadvantages:

> ❝It didn't last long. After a while I thought, this is quite nice, you know, no-one hogging the bathroom and if you decide you want to go off and do something, you don't have to worry about cooking for anyone or leaving food for them. So the feeling of loss did wear off quite quickly [laughs]. It was that all of a sudden his room was empty and I thought, arrrrr, oh dear.❞

Whilst much has been made of what is often termed, the 'empty nest syndrome', the majority of women adjust very well to the changes brought about when children leave home. Where there are a number of role changes, however, women may find it takes longer to adjust.

Death of family or friends

In addition to losing elderly relatives, women often have to face up to the death of friends and family members of a similar age to them. While the loss of a loved one can be emotionally distressing in itself, when the person is of a similar age, it can have an additional effect of increasing the awareness of a person's own mortality:

> ❝And seeing others go [die] makes you think of your own mortality or lack of immortality .... Because it seems so much nearer. It's like being on a conveyor belt and jogging along.❞

The feeling of loneliness after members of the family die can be particularly difficult to deal with during the middle years when a number of deaths may occur within a short time. Many women will have two parents and two parents-in-law who will be reaching the end of their lifetimes at a similar time:

> ❝My mother has recently died, and so that just leaves me now ... it seems a bit lonely when you think about it like that.❞

Such a sense of loneliness, brought about by the death of friends and family members, often occurs at the same time that women are making adjustments to children leaving home and the move towards retirement, or indeed a return to paid employment. While these changes may be manageable in isolation, women may find them more stressful when they occur in a short space of time.

Changes in relationships

The possible combined effect of the many changes arising during the middle years on relationships is complex. For example, what effect does the changing relationships with children have on relationships between husband and wife or partners? What is the impact of an increased awareness of mortality? What happens to a relationship when women are consumed by the responsibility of caring for elderly relatives as well as for children? Possibly as a result of these and other changes, women may experience a breakdown in their relationship with husbands or partners. Whilst this may be viewed negatively by some women, for others a move away from a long-term relationship can be seen as part of a much broader need to live the rest of their life in a different way. The last section of this chapter considers this within the context of women's changing outlook on life.

Changes in body image

Within Western societies, the menopause tends to be associated with ageing. This image appears to have been shaped by a number of factors. For example, as discussed in Chapter 1, there are a number of biological changes, such as dryer skin, brittle nails, changing fat distribution, and softer breasts, which occur when levels of oestrogen fall. In addition, women reach the menopause on average, at around the age of 50, which is often seen as a milestone age. The menopause also represents a change in a woman's ability to reproduce, and this is often associated with getting older. Unfortunately, within Western societies, there is also

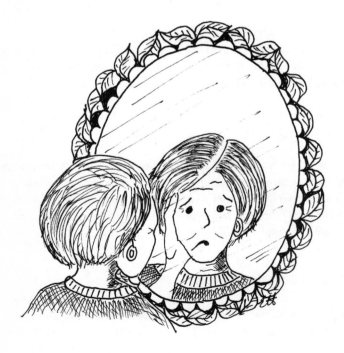

a tendency to view ageing negatively. For many women, therefore, the menopause is approached with concerns about ageing and a loss of value within society.

Most women notice changes in their physical appearance over their lifetime, but these changes are often more pronounced during the middle years. Many women find that they catch an unexpected glimpse of themselves in the mirror but find their mother's face staring back in the reflection. At first, this may be a bit alarming:

> **“**I must admit that the worse thing that I find is sometimes catching a glimpse of yourself unaware and you think, 'Oh dear' [laughs]. I was walking past a mirror the other day and I thought, 'Oh it's my mum!' And then I realised that it was me! [laughs].**”**

Although such a mirrored image is often initially disturbing, it is generally considered to be an inevitable part of ageing. Indeed, most of the women interviewed, spoke about their changing looks as part and parcel of life and something that was going to happen whatever they did. They often remarked that looking older was simply something that you had to come to terms with. In addition to looking older themselves, women often pointed out that their husband, partner or relative was also ageing. This sometimes allowed women to see themselves as ageing well, when compared to others of a similar age:

> **“**Well, I look in the mirror sometimes and I think, 'Oh girl, you are getting old'. But then I saw my sister-in-law the other day. I hadn't seen her for years ... she's the same age as me. And when I came home, I looked in the mirror and thought, 'You're not doing so bad after all' [laughs]. As you can see, my hair is going but that doesn't bother me. My eldest daughter is the only one who comments about it. She says, 'Why don't you colour your hair mum?' And I say, 'No, I'm quite happy'.**”**

As this woman says, the pressure on women to preserve their youthful looks can be generated from other people. This is largely because there is a tendency, within Western societies, to promote youthful women in a positive light and older women in a negative light. In other countries, such as China and Japan, where a higher status is awarded to women as they get older, the menopause is associated with fewer emotional symptoms than it is in Western societies.

Thus, in countries such as Britain and the USA, both the film and the advertising industries not only focus on youthful, glamorous images of women, but also encourage women to participate in age-resisting practices. A glance at the shelves of any high-street chemist shop will reveal that the number of anti-wrinkle creams for women far outweighs the number available for men.

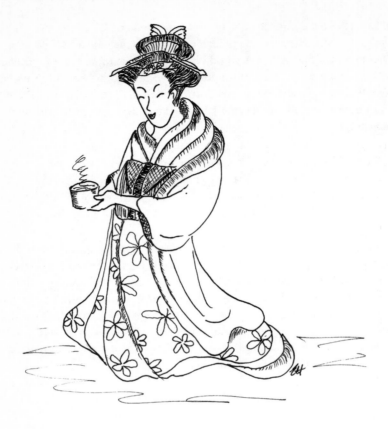

Although the majority of women interviewed said that they had accepted their ageing body image, for a few women, this was an area of concern:

> **❝**The thing that you see in the media very much is that your skin will get dehydrated and you will get wrinkles and errm you won't be sexually attractive. This is the way they're putting it. And you do start thinking, hmmm yes, well when you get to 40 or so, men stop looking at you. Maybe they're right. So I think you become a bit aware of that. For me I want to keep looking nice for as long as I can.**❞**

However, despite the focus on maintaining youthful looks within Western societies, most women expressed a greater concern about the possible changes in body function, rather than in body image. They spoke about their concerns about not being able to care for themselves when they got older and how physical disabilities would affect their quality of life in old age. Such images of physical deterioration are often influenced by women's experiences of caring for elderly relatives:

❝I don't like the thought of getting to a stage where I am not able to do what I want ... where you get to an age whereby you are bound by your physical constraints. And being a burden as they say ... When my aunt was taken into care I used to go and see her and see them all sitting around in this room and just staring into space and I thought, 'Oh I hope this is not in store for me'. That sort of thing worries me about old age. Not the getting old but the being incapacitated.**❞**

In addition to observing physical deterioration in elderly relatives, women may experience a number of subtle changes in their own health, many of which they recognise as marking the start of future disablement. The need for reading glasses, being unable to run for a bus, increased tiredness, or a general feeling that the body is slowing down, can all be reminders of an ageing body:

❝I think the body is getting slower. As I come to do that digging in the garden, I think it's all starting to slow a bit.**❞**

Although there are biological reasons linked to women's changing body image over the time of the menopause, the interview data collected in the *Women's Health Study* illustrates that these physical changes are influenced by social changes. The low value that older women have in Western societies, as well as exposure to elderly relatives who require care, both contribute to the idea that going through the menopause represents a stage in getting old.

A change in outlook on life

It is difficult to pinpoint what it is that brings many women to change their outlook on life during the middle years. A recent study carried out in Germany revealed that around half of menopausal women re-evaluated their life as a result of the menopause. Is it really the menopause that initiates women to consider their past life and re-think their future? Or do certain social changes provoke such a re-evaluation? In fact, it is unlikely to be just one factor that makes women re-think their position but, rather, a combination of a number of factors, many of which have been discussed in this chapter already. At some point, however, during the middle years, women seem to 'take stock' of their lives:

❝Because I sort of reached a point in my life where I was reassessing where I am going for the next few years. And it's happened to so many friends and people that I know at work as well. Ermmm ... so I think it's all part of a process really of working out things .... You suddenly take stock of what's happened so far. And it can be quite a sort of challenging time. Ermm, I was talking to a friend on Sunday who was going exactly through this, she's just a little bit older than me but she's feeling very depressed at the moment and can't quite see her way forward. I think I was probably at that kind of point about a year ago and I feel better now. Suddenly, you have to re-find your purpose again somehow I think. **99**

For many women, children often leave home around the time of the menopause, and this often brings about a change in role for women. This can be an important factor in bringing about a changed outlook in life, especially for women who have remained at home to look after the family and home. However, the impact of children leaving home on a woman's outlook on life varies, with some women seeing it as a time for new challenges, while others are struggling to find fulfilment in life.

For many women, reaching the age of 50 years provokes a re-evaluation of life. While they often see the age of 50 as a landmark for old age, on the whole there is a sense of inevitability with ageing and, therefore, it is not generally viewed negatively. Instead, when reaching the age of 50, there is a tendency to consider how the remaining years should be spent. Women often talk about having reached the half-way mark in life, and the way in which the rest of life is spent, therefore, needs some careful thought:

66Because you get to 50 and think, 'Well I'm half a century now. It's half a lifetime ... there are a lot more years left'. I think you need to be perhaps thinking of different things too do, different directions to take, things like that. **99**

Reaching the age of 50 years and realising that so much life has been spent already was disturbing for some women. This, however, does not generally last for very long and adjustments to being a person in their fifties are soon made:

66Well it did seem like a big milestone and I thought, 'Oh no, it's a downward slope from here on'. But I'm 53 now and I don't feel any different. Being 50 was a hiccup and I thought that this was it. But no, now I feel the same. **99**

In summary, women report a stage in their life where they feel the need to 'take stock' and re-evaluate where they are going and what they are doing. Although this is probably something that we all do to some extent throughout our lives, it seems a more prominent feature of middle age. At this time, in addition to the menopause, where biological changes are experienced, women have a number of other social changes. They reach the age of 50 years, they often have changes in social roles such as caring for elderly relatives or returning to paid employment, and they are faced with an increased illness and possibly death of friends and relatives. All these factors can contribute to what is probably aptly termed 'the change in life', where women may find themselves re-assessing the past and planning for their future. Although women can find this a time of unsettlement, this rarely lasts for long and usually results in a positive outlook for the future.

Summary

- A number of life changes may occur around the same time as the menopause and often have an impact on women's experiences of the menopause and their self-image.

- Life changes often result in women finding that they have to deal with a number of competing demands, for example, from elderly relatives, other family members and work.

- Employment changes in the form of return to paid employment, may offer women exciting new challenges, and subsequent increase in self-esteem. The transition to retirement from paid employment, whilst often seen as a positive change, may also alter the way in which a woman sees herself, especially when it comes at a time when children leave home.

- Although women experience life changes when children leave home, they mostly adjust to this with ease, finding that they benefit from increased independence.

- Most women notice changes in their physical appearance over their lifetime. Although these changes are often more pronounced during the middle years, the majority of women accept this changing image as an inevitable part of getting old.

- A change in outlook on life may be brought about by a number of social and cultural factors. For example, reaching the age of 50 years can lead women to 'take stock' of their life, often wanting to make the most of the years that remain. In addition, the loss of friends and family members of a similar age can increase women's awareness of their own mortality and raises questions about what the future holds.

Keeping healthy after the menopause

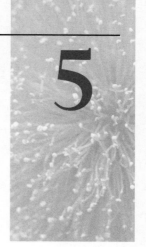

5

Oestrogen influences the structure and workings of many areas of the body. In particular, it has been shown to be protective against osteoporosis (brittle bone disease) and, to some extent, heart disease. In addition to the increased risk of osteoporosis and heart disease after the menopause, research has pointed towards a link between lowered oestrogen levels and the development of Alzheimer's disease. Each of these conditions will be discussed in turn within this chapter.

Osteoporosis

Osteoporosis, or brittle bone disease, occurs when there is a significant loss of bone mass and the bones become thin and vulnerable to being broken.

Although both men and women develop osteoporosis, men produce much greater levels of testosterone than women, which results in a higher peak bone mass and consequently, less chance of developing osteoporosis. In addition, after the age of around 35 years, the rate of bone loss is much faster in women than it is in men. In particular the rate of bone loss in women is accelerated at the time of the menopause, with up to 20 per cent of bone loss occurring in the first 10 years after menopause. The rate of bone loss slows thereafter. Thus, only one in twelve men over the age of 50 years will sustain a broken bone because of osteoporosis, compared with one in three women over the age of 50 years.

How do I know if I am at risk of osteoporosis?

There are no symptoms of osteoporosis and many women only find out that they have it when they break a bone. Although women considered to be at risk of osteoporosis are advised to have a bone scan, at present there is no universal policy

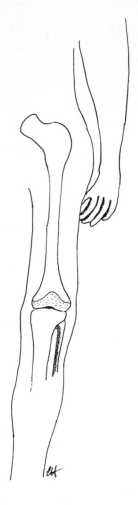

in the UK for widespread screening for the disease. Risk factors for osteoporosis are outlined in Box 5.

Box 5.	Women are at an increased risk of osteoporosis if they …

- Have a premature menopause (menopause occurs before the age of 40 years).

- Have a hysterectomy before the age of 40 years (this tends to result in an early menopause even when the ovaries are not removed). ▶

- Have a family history of osteoporosis.

- Have taken steroid therapy in the past for more than six months.

- Have had pre-menopausal absence of periods for longer than six months that was NOT due to pregnancy (may have been due to excessive dieting or exercising).

- Have a low body weight.

- Have liver or thyroid disease.

- Have a history of excessive alcohol intake.

- Smoke.

What happens during a bone scan?

Bone density can be calculated with the use of special equipment that measures the amount of radioactivity present in the bones. The test is generally carried out in hospital and usually takes up to an hour to complete. It is a completely non-invasive test, where a machine is passed slowly over the body. Many hospitals measure the density of just the hip and the backbone. There are no special preparations required prior to having the test, and normal activities can be resumed after the procedure has been completed.

How do I reduce my risks of osteoporosis?

For many women, osteoporosis can be easily prevented by a healthy lifestyle, including exercise and a balanced diet.

Box 6. Reducing the risks of osteoporosis.

For many women, the following self-help activities will be sufficient to protect against osteoporosis:

Self-help

- Increase dietary intake of calcium to 700 mg a day (see Box 7).

- Increase dietary intake of vitamin D to 400 IU a day (see Box 8).

- Take regular weight-bearing exercise such as brisk walking, keep-fit, tennis, aerobics, skipping and dancing. Try to exercise for 20 minutes, three times a week.

- Reduce alcohol consumption.

- Not smoking.

If you have been diagnosed as having osteoporosis or you are at particular risk of developing the disease (see Box 5), you may be advised to take one of the following therapies:

Drug therapy

- Calcium supplements to boost your calcium intake to 1200 mg per day.

- Hormone replacement therapy.

- Tibolone – a synthetic steroid with oestrogenic properties that help to prevent bone loss (see also Chapter 8).

- SERMs – a class of drugs that act on oestrogen receptors in the body and increase bone mass (see also Chapter 8).

- Bisphosphonates – drugs that help to prevent bone loss.

Alternative therapies

- Phyto-oestrogens (see Chapter 7 for more details).

- Natural progesterone (see Chapter 7 for more details).

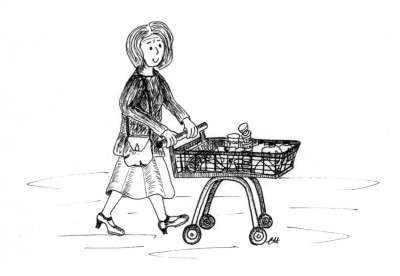

As stated in Box 6, the recommended daily intake of calcium for women is 700 mg a day. This can be achieved fairly simply by drinking one pint of milk each day. There are, however, a variety of other foods that also contain substantial amounts of calcium. Some examples are listed in Box 7.

Box 7.	Examples of foods rich in calcium.	
		Amount of calcium
Skimmed cow's milk	195 ml (1/3 pint)	250 mg
Semi-skimmed cow's milk	195 ml (1/3 pint)	240 mg
Natural yoghurt	140 g pot	270 mg
Cheddar cheese	50 g	400 mg
Edam cheese	50 g	370 mg
Salmon (tinned with bones)	100 g	195 mg
Sardines (tinned in oil)	100 g	460 mg
Tofu (soya bean curd)	100 g	507 mg
Red kidney beans	100 g	140 mg
White bread	2 large slices	60 mg
Wholemeal bread	2 large slices	14 mg
Broccoli	100 g	76 mg
Almonds	100 g	250 mg

In order that calcium can be properly absorbed by the body, adequate amounts of vitamin D need to be taken each day. The recommended daily intake of vitamin D for women is 400 IU per day and most people obtain this from a combination of diet and by being outside for part of the day in summer (sunshine provides a natural source of vitamin D). About 15–20 minutes of sunshine a day during the summer months allows the body to store adequate vitamin D supplies for the whole year. Many Asian women not only have a low dietary intake of vitamin D, but they also tend not to expose their skin to sunlight. These women are likely, therefore, to need vitamin D supplements.

Examples of foods rich in vitamin D are listed in Box 8.

Box 8.	Examples of foods rich in vitamin D.

- Margarine.
- Breakfast cereals.
- Oily fish, such as tuna.

▶

- Egg yolks.
- Liver.

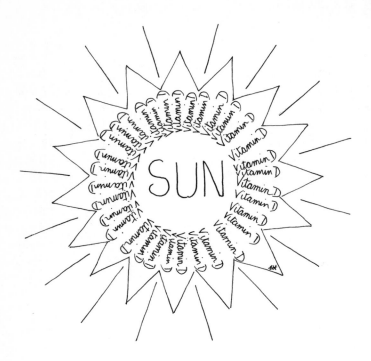

Although, for most women, osteoporosis can be prevented by a healthy diet and lifestyle, some women are at higher risk of developing the condition and may need to take drug therapy to prevent their bones from breaking.

Drug therapy for the prevention of osteoporosis

Since women experience an accelerated rate of bone loss at the time of the menopause, treatment needs to be started early in order to minimise bone loss. Oestrogen replacement therapy is generally the first treatment of choice, particularly as it has the added benefits of potentially providing symptom relief. In order to significantly reduce the incidence of broken bones, however, it has been suggested that HRT needs to be taken for at least 5–10 years. Once the therapy is stopped, the protective benefits against osteoporosis appear to be lost, although studies have yet to determine whether there is any residual protective effect from

HRT after discontinuation of use. The minimum daily dose for bone protection is: 2 mg of oestradiol valerate, 0.625 mg of conjugated oestrogens, and 50 mcg of transdermal oestradiol.

Although HRT needs to be taken on a long-term basis to maximise the protective benefits against osteoporosis, this increases the risks associated with the therapy. In particular, studies have shown that there is an increased risk of breast cancer associated with long-term use of HRT. This risk, however, does appear to be fairly small, and women need to weigh up the risk of osteoporosis against the risk of breast cancer (see also, Chapter 8).

HRT derivatives, such as tibolone and selective oestrogen receptor modulators (SERMs) have also been found to be beneficial in the prevention of osteoporosis. Some studies have shown up to 50 per cent reduction in bone fractures of the spine in women taking SERMs. The distinct advantage of SERMs is their ability to select the tissue sites that they act upon. They do not stimulate the breast tissue and are therefore able to reduce the risk of breast cancer associated with HRT. Research into the effectiveness of SERMs is ongoing, but it is hoped that they will be able to provide adequate protective benefits while not increasing the risk of breast cancer. See also Chapter 8.

Bisphosphonates, are a group of non-hormonal drugs, which have been found to be effective in preventing bone resorption and, therefore, bone loss. Etidronate and Alendronate are examples of those frequently prescribed. One of the key problems with bisphosphonates is that they are poorly absorbed through the stomach, and therefore have to be taken at least four hours after food. Since little is known about the long-term effects of bisphosphonates on the bone, they tend to be reserved for use in older women who have established osteoporosis. Younger women, who are at risk of osteoporosis, are generally advised to take HRT.

Calcium supplements may be advised for women who have been diagnosed as having osteoporosis and therefore need to have their total daily intake of calcium increased to 1200 mg per day. In addition, women who have a low dietary intake of calcium (less than 700 mg per day) may wish to take calcium supplements to help maintain healthy bones. Although they are not able to prevent bone loss, they do reduce the rate at which bone is lost.

Heart disease

Up until the time of the menopause heart disease is five times more common in men than in women. Following the menopause, however, women's risk of heart disease increases sharply, so that they have the same chances of experiencing heart disease as men. The mechanisms that increase women's risk of heart disease after the menopause are still not fully understood and research is ongoing in this area.

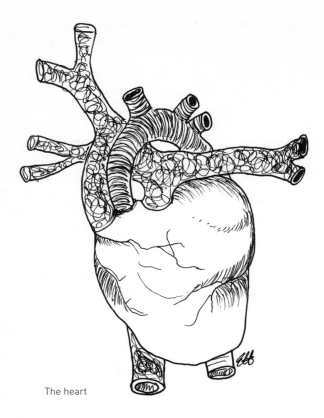

The heart

Studies suggest, however, that oestrogen has effects on the blood cholesterol level, the clotting mechanism, and the blood vessel walls. See also Chapter 1.

How do I know if I am at risk of heart disease?

As with osteoporosis, people tend to be unaware that they have heart disease until they experience symptoms. By this stage, however, the disease is fairly established. Box 9 outlines risk factors for heart disease.

Box 9.	Women are at increased risk of heart disease if they ...

- Have a family history of heart disease.

- Have high blood pressure.

- Have diabetes. ▶

- Experience a premature menopause (age forty or below).

- Smoke.

- Have a high blood cholesterol level.

- Have type A personality (are very competitive, time-driven, hostile and hard driving).

- Are overweight.

- Live a sedentary lifestyle.

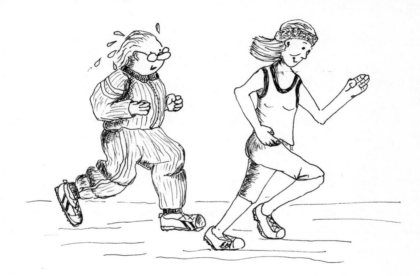

How can I reduce my risks of heart disease?

There are a number of ways in which the risk of heart disease can be reduced. These are outlined in Box 10.

Box 10. Reducing the risks of heart disease.

Self-help

- Maintain a low cholesterol diet – reduce intake of butter and red meat.

- Increase dietary intake of antioxidants, found in fresh fruit and vegetables and, in particular, in tomatoes.

- Ensure a good dietary intake of fibre (20–35 g per day), by eating foods such as wholegrain bread, oatmeal, brown rice, apples (with skin), oranges.

- Reduce weight if necessary.

- Stop smoking.

- Reduce stress.

- Exercise regularly.

Drug therapies

- Control blood pressure with anti-hypertensive drugs if necessary.

- A group of drugs called statins may be helpful in reducing a particularly high blood cholesterol.

- Oestrogen replacement therapy may be protective against heart disease. Oestrogen PLUS progesterone, however, is not recommended for the prevention of heart disease.

Alternative therapies

- Phyto-oestrogens (see Chapter 7 for more details).

Dietary and lifestyle changes for the prevention of heart disease

Although it is not possible to change a family or genetic tendency to heart disease, there are a number of dietary and lifestyle changes that can be made in order to minimise the chances of getting heart disease. In particular, smoking significantly increases the risk of heart disease, and so women who smoke are urged to give up. A lack of physical activity has also been found to increase the risk of heart disease. Studies indicate that approximately 30 minutes of moderate exercise a day, such as walking, dancing or gardening, will help to maintain a healthy heart.

A well-balanced diet, which is low in cholesterol and high in fibre, will help to reduce the risk of heart disease. The following dietary advice will help to maintain a healthy heart:

- **Fruits and vegetables** – Studies suggest that eating at least five portions of fruit and vegetables a day will provide a good source of antioxidants, which help to prevent furring up (atheroma) of the inside walls of the coronary arteries.

- **Fats and cholesterol** – Reducing the total dietary intake of fat will reduce the amount of fats in the blood. In addition to this, replacing some saturated fats with polyunsaturated fats and monounsaturated fats will help to improve the ratio of 'protective' cholesterol to 'harmful' cholesterol in your blood. Examples of foods containing saturated fats are: meats, full-fat dairy foods, and some vegetable oils such as coconut. Examples of polyunsaturated fats are: vegetable oils such as sunflower, corn and soya, and oily fish such as mackerel and sardine. Examples of monounsaturated fats are: olive and rapeseed oils, avocado pears, and nuts.

- **Fibre** – Studies suggest that eating a high-fibre diet may help to reduce the amount of cholesterol that the body absorbs into the bloodstream. Oats are high in soluble fibre, which is easily absorbed during digestion.

- **Fish and fish oils** – Eating oily fish regularly appears to help reduce the development of heart disease and also to improve the chances of survival after a heart attack. The exact mechanism by which this works is unknown, although research is currently being carried out in this area. It has, however, been suggested that fish oils help to keep the heartbeat regular, they reduce the level of triglycerides (fatty substances found in the blood), and they prevent blood clots from forming in the coronary arteries.

- **Salt** – A reduction in the amount of salt in the diet helps to keep the blood pressure down.

- **Alcohol** – Too much alcohol can damage the heart muscle and increase the blood pressure. In addition, excessive alcohol can lead to weight gain. However, moderate drinking (between one and two units of alcohol a day) can help protect the heart. One unit of alcohol is equal to either, one glass of wine, half-a-pint of ordinary beer, or one measure of spirit.

Drug therapy for the prevention of heart disease

The early treatment of high blood pressure or diabetes is important in the prevention of heart disease and, therefore, women with a family history of these diseases are advised to have regular health checks. In addition, women found to have a high blood cholesterol level may be advised to take statins (blood cholesterol reducing drugs).

Although some studies have shown that the prolonged use of oestrogen is associated with a 30–50 per cent reduction in heart disease, progesterone has been shown to significantly reduce the beneficial effects of oestrogen on the heart.[1] Indeed, a large American study, which was discontinued in 2002, when a greater proportion of women in the HRT group, compared with the non-HRT group, developed breast cancer, showed that oestrogen and progestin (a form of progesterone), when taken together, increased the risk of heart disease. The increased risk of heart disease, however, was very slight, being equal to seven more heart disease events occurring every year in 10 000 women taking oestrogen and progestin, when compared with women not taking HRT. This study (the Women's Health Initiative) concluded that the HRT being tested (a combination of continuous oestrogen and progestin) 'should not be initiated or continued for primary prevention of coronary heart disease'.

Although the Women's Health Initiative (WHI) had to discontinue the HRT study that used oestrogen and progestin, they were able to continue a parallel study where an oestrogen-only treatment is being used. The results of this study, which are due to be released in 2005 may well reveal that oestrogen alone is protective against heart disease. As indicated earlier, however, where a woman has not had a hysterectomy, progesterone is needed to minimise the risk of endometrial cancer.

The WHI finding that oestrogen and progestin increases the risk of heart disease, reflects the results of an earlier American study, the Heart and Estrogen/Progestin Replacement Study (HERS), where women with heart disease were found to have an increased risk of further heart disease when taking oestrogen and progestin.

Alzheimer's disease

Alzheimer's disease is a condition characterised by a progressive deterioration in cognition (the ability of the brain to carry out thought processes), with a gradual loss of memory and a loss of control over the body. In the early stages of Alzheimer's disease, there is a tendency towards forgetfulness and an increasing inability to find the right words. In the very late stages of the disease, the ability to talk often disappears altogether and the brain appears to be unable to tell the body what to do. The risk of Alzheimer's disease increases as a person gets older, with 15 per cent of people in their eighties developing the condition.

Although both men and women develop Alzheimer's disease, recent research has shown that the body's oestrogen is important for the maintenance of healthy tissue in specific parts of the brain. In particular, oestrogen is required in the part of the brain that is responsible for memory. Studies have shown that there is a lower incidence of Alzheimer's disease in women who take hormone replacement therapy. Moreover, those women who do develop Alzheimer's disease, but take

---

[1] Since oestrogen has been found to increase the risk of endometrial cancer (cancer of the lining of the womb), women who wish to take HRT, and have not had a hysterectomy, need to take progesterone in order to minimise the risk of endometrial cancer.

HRT, are generally found to have a milder form of the disease. So it has been suggested that HRT may not only offer treatment possibilities for Alzheimer's disease, but may also be useful for protection against age-related brain tissue loss. Research into this area is ongoing.

It has been suggested that there are some possible risk factors for Alzheimer's disease, although, once again, further research needs to be carried out to determine the precise nature of the risks. Possible risk factors are:

- A family history of Alzheimer's disease.
- Head injury.
- Menopause.
- Depression.
- Low thyroid function.

It has also been suggested that it may be possible to reduce the risk of Alzheimer's disease. In addition to hormone replacement therapy, smoking and the long-term use of non-steroidal anti-inflammatory drugs appear to offer some protection against Alzheimer's disease. Further research in this area, however, is needed.

Summary

- The chance of developing osteoporosis increases after the menopause when the rate of bone loss accelerates. For many women, osteoporosis can be prevented by a healthy lifestyle, including exercise and a balanced diet.

- Some women are at particular risk of developing osteoporosis and may be advised to take therapies such as HRT or bisphosphonates to help reduce their risk of broken bones.

- Although the body's own oestrogen is protective against heart disease, after the menopause, when oestrogen levels fall, women's risk of heart disease increases so that it matches that experienced by men. Lifestyle changes such as stopping smoking, keeping physically fit and eating a well-balanced diet, which is low in fat and high in fibre, will contribute to a reduced risk of heart disease.

- Studies suggest that oestrogen therapy, when taken on its own (i.e. not in combination with progesterone), reduces the risk of heart disease. However, when taken in combination with progesterone, research has shown that women experience an increased risk of heart disease.

● The body's own oestrogen appears to provide women with some protection against Alzheimer's disease. Research suggests that hormone replacement therapy may be useful in the treatment and prevention of Alzheimer's disease. Further research is required in this area.

Changes in the menopause over time

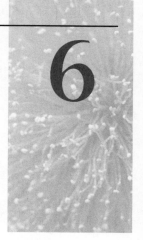

6

Although today we understand the menopause as occurring when there is a decline in oestrogen production, knowledge about the female reproductive system, and consequently, the menopause, has evolved over time. This chapter will describe the changing ways in which the menopause has been understood over time, and the treatments that have been used over the years.

Ways of understanding and treating the menopause have developed over the years. Although in the ancient world many women did not live long enough to experience the menopause, around one-third of women reached the age of 50 years, and therefore will have had some similar experiences to women of today.

In the ancient world, scientists such as Hippocrates, Aristotle and Galen based their understanding of human anatomy and physiology on what was termed 'humoral theory'. At this time, the body was thought to contain four fluids called 'humors', which needed to be kept in balance to ensure good health. Blood was seen as one of these humors, and good health relied on the right amount of blood being kept in the body. A variety of illnesses, experienced by both men and women were believed to be caused by an excess of blood in the body. Removal of blood was therefore seen as a way of cleansing the body from the toxic effects of blood. Although women got rid of excess blood through menstruation, men had to have it removed through a process of bloodletting, where blood was drawn from the veins in the arms or legs.

When women ceased to menstruate at the menopause, the symptoms they experienced were believed to arise from an excess of blood being retained in the body. Treatment was therefore based on removing blood using a variety of methods.

The earliest record of treatments for the menopause, or as it was then called, 'the cessation of menses', can be found in a book called *The Diseases of Women* written in the eleventh century, by Trotula di Ruggiero, a female 'doctor for women'. Trotula believed that menstruation ceased because blood became trapped within the abdomen. In order to restore the body's balance of blood, Trotula recommended lancing the vein in the foot and drawing one pint of blood from alternate feet each

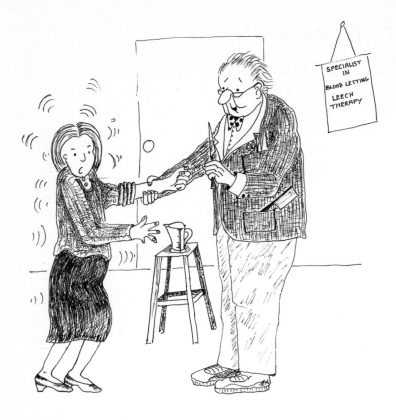

day. Blood was also removed by applying leeches to the cervix, where they would suck out trapped blood directly from the womb. In addition to this, medicine to relieve constipation was recommended, as this was thought to contribute to the blood being trapped inside the body.

As well as trying to remove trapped blood from within the body, Trotula advised a variety of treatments for restoring menstruation. Treatments included, bathing regularly and drinking a mixture of 'calamento', catnip or mint, cooked with honey. Women were also advised to drink this herbal mixture in the bath, or to infuse the herbs into the bathwater. In addition, steam was administered directly to the womb by getting women to sit over a boiling pot of catnip, covered with a perforated gall bladder from a bull. If necessary, a reed or a tube was inserted into the vagina and used to direct the steam. Diuretics such as fennel or parsley were also thought to be helpful, as was a mixture of wormwood, skirtwood, saliva, wild marjoram, nettle, honey, pennyroyal, privet and dill, which was cooked and applied to the abdomen. If all of these remedies failed, Trotula recommended that a mixture of powdered soda, the gall bladder of a bull and the juice of parsley were soaked into shredded wool and then inserted into the vagina.

The idea that the menopause was caused by blood being trapped within the body continued through to the mid-nineteenth century. By this time, an increasing number of symptoms were attributed to what was believed to be the toxic effects of retained blood. Symptoms included flushing, headaches, restlessness, anxiety, troublesome dreams, unequal spirits, inflammation of the bowels or other internal parts, spasmodic affections of various parts, stiffness of the limbs, swollen ankles, piles and other effects of plenitude. Treatment of these symptoms did not differ much from those recommended by Trotula back in the eleventh century and focused largely on frequent removal of blood, keeping the bowels lax and moderating women's diet.

Doctors also advised women to drink several glasses of effervescing lemonade over the course of the day, to eat meat once a day, and to avoid beer or porter, taking for preference one glass of sherry at dinner. In addition, it was suggested that women should bath for one hour every week and exercise more in the open air.

By the nineteenth century, knowledge grew about the structure of the ovary and its functions, and in 1821 doctors started to use the term 'menopause' to describe the cessation of menstruation. Over the mid- to late-nineteenth century, rather than seeing menopausal symptoms as resulting from the toxic effects of trapped blood, some form of irregular activity of the nervous system was believed to be responsible for changes in ovarian function. While little was known about the substance 'oestrogen', the ovary was believed to produce 'juices', and during the menopause, the nervous system was thought to reduce the amount of ovarian juices being produced. A reduction of ovarian juices was also believed to result in diseased ovaries, which in turn, was thought to have some reaction upon the general nervous system. Hence, the association between the menopause and the nervous system was established.

Possibly drawing on the link between the ovaries and the nervous system, many of the medical books written from the mid-nineteenth century onwards described the menopause as a time of great psychological disturbance for women. Indeed one of the most frequently cited symptoms of the menopause was reported to be nervous irritability, with some doctors suggesting that almost all menopausal women experienced this symptom. Thus, in the 1850s, a study by a British physician, Edward Tilt, reported that out of a sample of 500 menopausal women, 459 suffered with nervous irritability, 208 suffered with headache, 146 from a hysterical state and 16 from insanity. However, working-class woman were believed to be less vulnerable to psychological disturbance associated with the menopause because, it was alleged, they did not have such sensitively organised nervous systems.

The idea that the ovary and the nervous system were inextricably linked, continued through the nineteenth century. Thus, in the 1870s, Robert Battey, a British surgeon, popularised an operation (oopherectomy) to remove the ovaries from women who were considered to be suffering from neurosis related to the ovary. It is believed that Battey removed one or both ovaries from some two or three thousand women thought to be suffering from ovarian-related nervousness. Indeed, the term 'to go batty', meaning to go mad, has its origins in Robert Battey's extensive surgery on women.

A number of less radical treatments were also available during the nineteenth century, although, once again, many focused on the treatment of a 'neurotic' disorder. Instead of baths being considered useful to release trapped blood from the body, as was the idea before the nineteenth century, they were prescribed for their sleep-enhancing properties. Substances such as mustard were added to the bathwater to induce sleep in the menopausal woman with nervous irritability.

By 1889 doctors were experimenting, both on themselves and on patients, with extracts of animal glands such as the ovaries, testes and the thyroid, and organs such as the heart and the brain. Both testicular and ovarian extracts were reported to combat many of the signs of old age and ovarian extracts were claimed to successfully treat women with 'insanity'. Although there was much controversy amongst doctors over the effectiveness of ovarian extracts in the treatment of menopausal symptoms, over the next 20 years or so, a number of commercial companies produced organ extracts and sold them directly to women. The ovaries of cows were mainly used, although those obtained from sows were also thought to be beneficial. Treatment usually involved ingestion of either fresh or dried animal ovary, eight or nine times a day for about one month, the effects being thought to last for 3 to 4 months.

In addition to being used for the treatment of menopausal symptoms, ovarian extracts were promoted for their ability to maintain youth. As Hancock & Co. stated on a pamphlet advertising ovarian extracts in 1930: 'Youth lasts as long as the glandular system is properly nourished and stimulated'. Thus, the link between the ovaries and a youthful appearance was made.

Having found that ovarian tissue was helpful in the relief of menopausal symptoms, in 1923 two British scientists, Allen and Doisy, reported their work on the localisation and extraction of the ovarian hormone, which they named 'oestrus'. Following this, oestrogenic treatments were derived from the amniotic fluid of cattle. By 1938, Diethylstilbestrol, a synthetic oral oestrogen treatment, had been developed and, within 1 year, 21 British companies made or imported natural and synthetic hormones. A few years later, Premarin®, an oestrogen preparation derived from the urine of pregnant mares, was developed.

Over the following twenty years or so, these oestrogen preparations were promoted by the pharmaceutical industry for their ability to relieve menopausal symptoms. Following the trend set in the late-nineteenth century, the main symptoms associated with the menopause related to psychological disturbances.

The menopause was portrayed as a traumatic experience, inevitably requiring medical treatment, which aimed to help women come to terms with what was seen as an 'identity crisis'. Advertisements for oestrogen treatments placed in medical journals used images such as melancholic, menopausal women, broken crockery and ships in a storm. However, this occurred amidst a more general increasing awareness about the potential for human emotional vulnerability, as well as new developments in psychiatric drugs. The use of testosterone for treating what had been termed the 'male climacteric' also grew in popularity at this time. Like women, men were seen as suffering from depression and nervous instability during their middle years.

Such was the perceived severity of women's emotional distress during the menopause that pharmaceutical companies manufactured combined oestrogen and sedative drug preparations. In addition, sedative drugs containing phenobarbitone and belladonna, which acts in a similar way to Valium® (a once popularly prescribed drug to relieve anxiety), were recommended for treating women during the menopause. In addition to oestrogen and sedatives, menopausal treatments included restriction of the daily calorie intake, a brisk walk in the fresh air once a day, a daily hot bath, exposure to artificial sunlight, Turkish baths, body massage and medication to keep the bowels open.

In 1966, an American doctor, Robert Wilson, published what came to be a very influential book called *Feminine Forever*. In this book, Wilson suggested that the menopause was an 'oestrogen deficiency' disease, which required continuous treatment with oestrogen therapy. There was, however, much criticism about Wilson's claims, especially amongst feminist writers. Thus, during the 1960s and 1970s, the idea that all women experiencing the menopause were emotionally fragile was criticised, and with the rise of second-wave feminism at this time, medical treatment of the menopause was contested.

Despite this resistance against the widespread treatment of menopausal symptoms, oestrogen had been found to be useful, firstly in the treatment and subsequently the prevention, of osteoporosis. Thus, by the late 1970s, some doctors were suggesting that after the menopause, *all* women might benefit from taking oestrogen on a long-term basis to protect them against osteoporosis. More recently oestrogen has been found to have potentially protective properties in the prevention of coronary heart disease and possibly Alzheimer's disease. However, much of the research into these two latter preventive uses of oestrogen is ongoing, and conclusions have yet to be reached. See Chapter 5 for discussions about the use of hormone replacement therapy for the prevention of diseases.

Although oestrogen appeared to offer many benefits, not only for the relief of menopausal symptoms, but also for the prevention of disease, during the 1970s doctors found that women taking oestrogen were more likely to develop cancer of the endometrium (lining of the womb). Over the following few years, however, research showed that the endometrium could be protected by giving oestrogen in combination with progesterone. Thus, women who had not had a hysterectomy were given 5–7 days of progesterone per month, in addition to the oestrogen. This combined treatment became known as 'opposed oestrogen therapy', compared with oestrogen-only preparations, which were termed 'unopposed oestrogen therapy'. It was also around this time that hormone treatments came to be known as 'hormone replacement therapy' or 'HRT'.

During the late 1970s and 1980s it was becoming apparent that as well as the risk of endometrial cancer, there might be a relationship between HRT and breast cancer. Numerous studies were then carried out over the next 20 to 30 years to determine the pros and cons of HRT. In 1997, a research group re-analysed the results of over 50 studies and concluded that women taking HRT were at a slight increased risk of breast cancer, especially when taking the therapy for a number of years. These findings were confirmed by the results of a large American study (Women's Health Initiative) reporting in 2002, which showed that after 4 years of taking continuous oestrogen and a form of progesterone, women were more likely to get breast cancer than those not taking the therapy. The study showed that for every 10 000 women taking oestrogen and progesterone each year, compared with those not taking it, there would be an additional eight women who would get breast cancer. This same study also reported that for every 10 000 women taking oestrogen and progesterone each year, compared with those not taking it, seven more women would have a heart attack, eight more would have a stroke, and eight more would have a blood clot. However, the study also showed that there would be six fewer bowel cancers and five fewer broken hips per year in every 10 000 women taking the therapy. See also Chapter 8 for further details on the risks and benefits associated with HRT.

Research into the pros and cons of HRT continue, with large national trials currently being undertaken in the United States and the United Kingdom. See Chapter 10 for further details of current research studies.

Summary

- In the ancient world, doctors believed that women ceased to menstruate in the middle years when blood became trapped within the body. Treatment of symptoms, therefore, concentrated on different ways of removing the trapped blood.

- The menopause got its name in 1821, when medical knowledge about the function of the ovaries increased. However, oestrogen was not actually identified until the early 1900s.

- During the nineteenth century, many doctors believed that the function of the ovaries was linked to the nervous system. Women were often identified as being emotionally unstable during the menopause, and treatments, therefore, were aimed at reducing women's 'nervous irritability'.

- The first synthetic oestrogen preparations were developed in the 1930s and were promoted by the pharmaceutical industry for the relief of menopausal symptoms.

- From the 1970s onwards, hormone replacement therapy has been promoted, not only for symptom relief, but also for the prevention of osteoporosis and heart disease. The risks and benefits associated with HRT have been, and continue to be, investigated.

- HRT in the form of continuous oestrogen plus a type of progesterone has been found to increase the chances of getting breast cancer, heart disease, blood clots, and strokes, but decrease the chances of getting osteoporosis and bowel cancer.

Non-hormonal therapies for the menopause

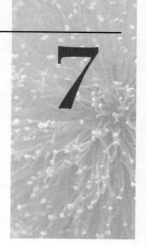

Not all women will require, or wish to take, treatments for the menopause. However, where symptom relief or long-term protection from diseases such as osteoporosis is required, women may wish to choose from a range of non-hormonal and hormonal therapies.

One of the major problems in trying to present an unbiased view about various menopausal treatments is that there is a lack of clear evidence surrounding the value of 'non-hormonal' therapies. This is largely because, in the past, the pharmaceutical industry has invested a great deal of money into developing and researching the effects of HRT, and there has been a lack of money invested in the development of non-hormonal therapies. More recently, however, there has been an increased interest in the potential value of non-hormonal therapies, with a growing number of studies being carried out in this area.

This chapter focuses on some of the popular non-hormonal therapies available for the menopause, and the following chapter focuses on hormonal treatments.

Isoflavones

Isoflavones are water-soluble chemicals that are found in many plants. One group of isoflavones is called phyto-oestrogens, which have similar effects in the body to those of oestrogen. Much of the research into the effects of phyto-oestrogen isoflavones concerns those that are found in soya products.

Although phyto-oestrogens are less powerful than the body's own oestrogen, they latch on to the same places (receptor sites) in the cells as oestrogen does. Studies have shown that phyto-oestrogens significantly reduce the severity of hot flushes, although not necessarily the frequency of flushes. In addition, recent research indicates that phyto-oestrogens may reduce the risk of both osteoporosis and heart disease.

89

Foods that are high in phyto-oestrogens include, roasted soya beans, tempeh (fermented soya beans), soya flour, and processed soya products such as soya protein and soya milk. In addition, green split peas, chick peas and broad beans are rich in some isoflavones. Isoflavones can also be purchased in tablet form from large high-street chemists.

Red clover (*Trifolium pratense*)

The same phyto-oestrogens found in soya are also contained in the herb, red clover, which is available in tablet form. This herb has been traditionally used to treat whooping cough, gout and cancer, although there is little evidence to support these uses.

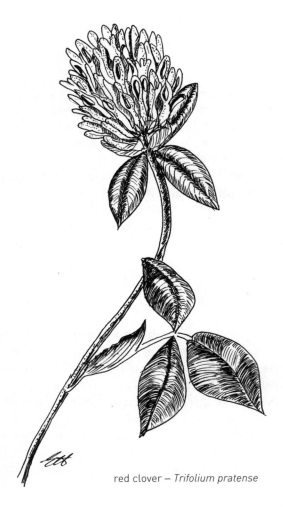

red clover — *Trifolium pratense*

A great deal of research has, however, been carried out on the use of red clover during and after the menopause. Studies suggest that, in addition to being effective in the reduction of hot flushes, red clover increases bone density, and should therefore reduce the risk of osteoporosis. Red clover also appears to improve cardiovascular function in post-menopausal women by increasing the elasticity of the blood vessels and reducing the cholesterol levels in the blood. Little is known about any possible long-term problems associated with phyto-oestrogens.

Possible drug interactions: red clover has been reported to increase the effects of an anti-clotting drug, called warfarin.

Wild yam

A yam is a root vegetable that resembles a large potato, and comes from the root of tropical vines. Various species of wild yam grow throughout North and Central America and Asia. Traditionally, this plant has been used as a treatment for indigestion, coughs, morning sickness, gall bladder pain menstrual cramps, joint pain and nerve pain.

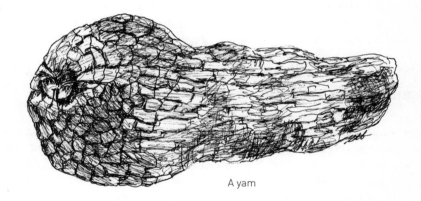

A yam

It has also been suggested that extracts of wild yam have oestrogenic and progestogenic properties, and can therefore be useful for the relief of menopausal symptoms and for the prevention of osteoporosis. To date, however, studies have shown that both the natural oestrogenic and progestogenic properties of yams are only effective in animals. When used in humans, therefore, progesterone has to be chemically transformed from the substance, diosgenin, which is contained in yams. Extracts of yam can be applied topically to the skin in the form of a cream, and manufacturers promote them as a 'natural HRT'. Since the progesterone has to be manufactured from the wild yam, however, the term 'natural progesterone' or 'natural HRT' is not strictly correct.

In addition, the evidence to support the effectiveness of yams is weak, with a number of studies showing little or no improvement in symptom relief or in bone mass. A possible reason for this apparent lack of efficacy is that the amount of yam extract being used is not large enough to provide adequate oestrogenic and progestogenic effects.

St John's wort

When taken internally, this plant has a relaxing action on the nervous system and can be useful in mild to moderate depression. Recent research has shown St John's wort to be as effective as certain antidepressant drugs in improving mood. An added advantage of St John's wort is that it was also found to be related with fewer side-effects than conventional antidepressant drug therapy. Nevertheless, side-effects associated with St John's wort include, dry mouth, dizziness, gastric irritation and fatigue.

Possible drug interactions: St John's wort has effects on enzymes found in both the liver and bowel, and may cause interactions with drugs such as anti-clotting agents, antidepressants, anti-epileptic drugs, anti-viral drugs, barbiturates, some heart drugs, oestrogens and progestogens. In addition, St John's wort may be associated with hair loss.

Agnus-castus (chasteberry)

Agnus-castus is a shrub in the verbena family and is commonly found on river banks and nearby foothills in central Asia and around the Mediterranean Sea. As the name 'chasteberry' implies, for centuries it was thought to reduce sexual desire and was drunk by the Romans to diminish libido. In ancient Greece, young women celebrating the festival of Demeter wore chasteberry blossoms to show that they were remaining chaste in honour of the goddess. Monks in the Middle Ages also used the fruit to reduce libido and it is from this that the name 'monk's pepper' originates.

Most studies have focused on the use of agnus-castus in the treatment of premenstrual symptoms, and in particular, its ability to relieve breast tenderness. However, women have also reported its usefulness in the relief of menopausal symptoms, although there is no real evidence to support its effectiveness. There do not appear to be any adverse reactions with agnus-castus.

Black cohosh

Black cohosh is a tall perennial herb originally found in the United States, which has mild oestrogenic properties. Native Americans used it mainly for women's health problems, but also as a treatment for arthritis, fatigue, and snakebite. There are a few studies that suggest that black cohosh may improve menopausal symptoms such as hot flushes, headache, heart palpitations, nervousness, irritability, sleep disturbance, anxiety, vaginal dryness, and depression. Although there is limited evidence, it would seem that black cohosh might function similarly to oestrogen in some tissues but not others. The herb has not, however, been shown to help prevent osteoporosis or heart disease. This is not to say that it will not provide some protection, but adequate investigation into this use of the plant has not been carried out.

Some women report headaches, weight gain, dizziness and gastric irritation when taking black cohosh.

Dong quai (*Angelica sinensis*)

Dong quai is one of the major herbs used in Chinese medicine. Traditionally, dong quai is said to be one of the most important herbs for strengthening the 'xue'. The Chinese term 'xue' is often translated as 'blood', but it actually refers to a more complicated set of ideas, of which the blood itself is only a part. In the late 1800s, an extract of dong quai, became popular in Europe, and was referred to as a 'female tonic' and, in the West, this is how most people consider it in now.

Dong quai is often recommended as a treatment for menstrual cramps, pre-menstrual symptoms and menopausal symptoms such as hot flushes. However, there is little scientific evidence to support these uses.

Possible drug interactions: dong quai has been reported to increase the actions of the drug warfarin. Certain constituents of dong quai may cause increased sensitivity to the sun, but there do not appear to be any reports of this.

Evening primrose oil

Evening primrose oil provides a rich source of gamolenic acid, which has been reported by women to be effective in alleviating hot flushes. However, very few studies have been carried out to determine its effectiveness and research into this area would be helpful. A small study of 56 women, where half the group took

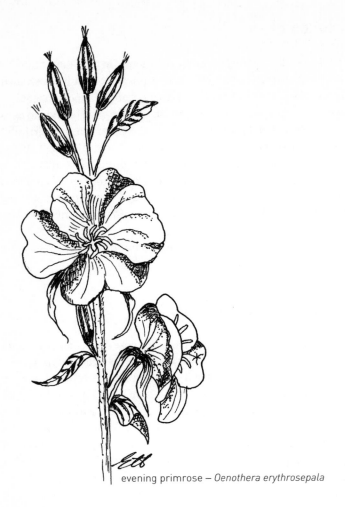

evening primrose – *Oenothera erythrosepala*

evening primrose oil and the other half took a substance that had no medicinal benefits (a placebo), showed no difference in the incidence of hot flushes between the two groups.

Capsules containing evening primrose oil are widely available from high-street chemist stores. Some women report nausea and diarrhoea when taking evening primrose oil.

Women's reported use of non-hormonal therapies

In the *Women's Health Study* survey, one-quarter of women stated that they had taken non-hormonal therapies for the relief of menopausal symptoms, the most popular being evening primrose oil. Other therapies included a variety of herbal remedies, Menopace, vitamins and homeopathic remedies.

The survey also showed that women with less severe menopausal symptoms tended to take non-hormonal therapies, whereas women with more severe symptoms tended to take HRT. This suggests that women prefer to take hormonal drugs only when really necessary and that non-hormonal therapies are reserved for less severe symptoms. Indeed, on the whole, the *Women's Health Study* interviews also reflected this use of non-hormonal therapies for milder symptoms:

> **"**I just don't think I feel bad enough to take HRT. I think with what I've done, taking the St John's wort, I've coped with it. Whereas if I really got to a bad state, then I think I might possibly consider it [HRT]. I'm not a very good person about taking pills and potions and things like that. I tend to think ... what is it? Physician heal yourself, sort of thing. I suppose if I was that poorly I think I would possibly try HRT. I would try other alternatives first and then if they didn't work, then I would maybe try HRT. **"**

The effectiveness of non-hormonal therapies varied greatly amongst the women, with some gaining great relief from menopausal symptoms, and others finding little improvement. Thus, for some women, evening primrose oil appeared to be effective in relieving symptoms:

> **"**And I've been taking evening primrose oil for a couple of years now. I started it when the hot flushes started being a nuisance. I remember that I had a temporary job in an office ... and I was absolutely burning [laughs] just flaming and perspiring. And I thought, I could do without this. And I battled along with it for about 2 or 3 months and so anyway, I started taking the evening primrose oil. It didn't work at once of course but after about 3 months I did notice that they [hot flushes] started lessening ... now whether they would have started lessening anyway I don't know. But I think it probably did help. **"**

Other women, however, found little, if any, relief from hot flushes when they took evening primrose oil:

> **"**When I started the menopause ... and had the hot flushes I took oil of evening primrose, which I took religiously for a year. And to be perfectly honest, ... I mean alright I don't know how I would have felt if I hadn't been taking it, but at the end of the year, I thought, 'Oh I can't see what good this is doing me', and so I left off and I didn't notice the difference. Errrrm as I say, I don't know how many flushes I would have got if I wasn't taking them.

But when I decided that I would stop them, I can't say that I really noticed any great fall off in my health or increase in any flushes or anything like that and so I didn't bother to take them again. **"**

Other non-hormonal therapies reported to be particularly effective in the relief of hot flushes, were black cohosh and wild yams:

"It's called black cohosh and wild yam. Brilliant stuff, absolutely brilliant. Worked for me a treat! Stopped the hot flushes. I mean you might just get a slight one every now and again, but it works brilliantly. I started with the maximum dose of three times a day as they said . . . . But I've never taken herbal remedies – not before I had the hot flushes. **"**

A combination of wild yams and agnus-castus was also reported to be effective in reducing hot flushes. Some treatments, however, were not always completely effective:

"I began to look for an alternative way, and I read about this wild yam cream and so I started taking agnus-castus and the wild yam cream about 10 days ago. And the hot flushes are much better. It *has* reduced the hot flushes – very much so. They haven't gone away but they are reduced and I feel better . . . . They occur [hot flushes] about three times in the day and none at night now, which is perfect. **"**

Phyto-oestrogens were also taken in the form of soya tablets, called soyagen. Again, some women reported these to be effective:

"I take the soyagen as well as natural progesterone. That is wonderful. I had hot flushes, but I haven't had any since I started taking the soyagen tablets. **"**

A further symptom being treated with non-hormonal therapies was a fall in libido (sex drive). Although few women had tried remedies for this, those who did, appeared to have found some relief:

"I saw a letter in the newspaper. It said, 'Since the menopause, I seemed to have lost every errrr . . . interest . . . in sex . . . is there any thing that can help?' And they recommended a Chinese thing, called angelica – angelica root. And errmm you take it as a liquid and you take 5 ml a day and they say that it improves everything. Chinese women take it as a tonic and it's supposed to improve every part of your body. So I thought, 'Oh great! We'll have a go at this'. And to be quite honest, I mean I know that it could all be in the mind but since I've started taking it, I really do feel better ... things have improved. And this is from about a fortnight after taking it. I have been taking it for about 6 weeks now. **"**

Treating emotional problems, such as anxiety or panicky feelings, largely involved the use of St John's wort, which women were able to buy from their local chemist shop. The few women who took St John's wort reported it to be effective in relieving their psychological symptoms:

"I started St John's wort ... I know it sounds stupid, but I started taking it leading up to my daughter's wedding because things, family-wise were getting a bit horrible. You know, family problems. And I was getting a bit stressed and having anxiety attacks.

But I think that it [St John's wort] actually did work. But then again, is it because you are taking something and psychologically you are thinking, 'Oh I must be better'. And then because I was coping so well for such a long time, I thought, well I'll take myself off of it. I think I stopped taking it 6–9 months ago. I must have taken it for about 18 months. But now I've started getting this sort of panicky feeling. I get like panicky about things. Well I'm calling them anxiety attacks but it's like ... like a feeling inside. I wake up with it, thinking, 'Oh God, I've got to do such and such today'. So I think I might go back on it again [laughs]. **"**

A frequently reported symptom that women associated with the menopause was aches and pains in joints. Many women reported taking cod liver oil over a number of years, in an effort to maintain healthy bones and to ease joint movements. Although it was not always possible to determine the effectiveness of the cod liver oil, largely because it was being taken for many years, most women believed that it was helpful:

"I've had the odd twinge in my fingers and I've just assumed that it's arthritis or something like that. In fact, I've been taking fish oil at night. I've been taking them for a long time now. Since taking them, I've found that my hands have been better. I just forget that I'm taking the fish oil. Whether it is just lubricating the joints, I don't know. It's only recently that I've noticed that the joints are getting better though. I took one type for a while and didn't notice a great deal of difference. But when I started taking this new one that I've been taking for quite a while now, I have definitely noticed an improvement. **"**

In addition to cod liver oil, seeds such as sunflower and sesame seeds were found to be effective in reducing joint pains:

❝I went to an exhibition and there was a stall up there that sold seeds ... and there were all these like poppy seeds, sesame seeds ... all these in a like toffee, crispy thing. So I bought a big pot and I ate the whole lot! [laughs]. All in a week, but it was absolutely delicious .... But all the pains in my ankles and knees disappeared. They just disappeared. And then somebody told me about this HRT cake, and she said, 'Why don't you try this? That's got all these seeds and soya milk and things in it.' So I decided to make it and I've been eating it every day, ever since [laughs]. And I've had no pains at all. Now whether this is just coincidence, I really don't know. But I'll have to wait and see, but I haven't left it off because I daren't, just in case the pains come back.❞

Although women often get some relief from non-hormonal therapies, some of the products on the market today can be fairly expensive. This will mean that many women will be unable to afford them, especially on a long-term basis:

❝Well I have looked at some of the alternative things, but they're so expensive. To be honest, they are so expensive that I couldn't afford to get myself hooked on them. I'd rather go and get a good hair-do or buy myself something nice to wear to cheer myself up than have to carry on paying all that kind of money out for them. And at the end of the day, who knows whether they really are as good as they say they are. But they are very, very expensive.❞

In addition to using non-hormonal therapies for the relief of menopausal symptoms, almost one-quarter of women in the survey took calcium tablets to help protect their bones against osteoporosis. As discussed in Chapter 5, it is advisable for women at particular risk of osteoporosis, or who have a low dietary intake of calcium (less than 700 mg per day), to take calcium supplements in order to protect their bones.

Summary

- Non-hormonal therapies such as evening primrose oil, agnus-castus, black cohosh and St John's wort, may provide relief from menopausal symptoms. In addition, research suggests that phyto-oestrogens, found in plants, appear to reduce the risk of osteoporosis and heart disease, as well as providing symptom-relief.

Further research into the effectiveness of non-hormonal therapies is needed.

● Around a quarter of women take non-hormonal therapies during the menopause. Their reports about the effectiveness of these therapies vary.

Hormonal treatments for the menopause

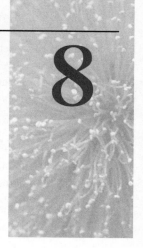

8

Hormone replacement therapy, popularly known as HRT, is the term used for the replacement of female hormones, oestrogen and progesterone, which decrease during the menopause transition. In other countries, such as the United States, it is usually referred to as 'estrogen replacement therapy' (ERT).

In addition, the male hormone, testosterone is sometimes given. Within this chapter, the use of these hormones, including the possible side-effects or complications associated with taking them, will be discussed.

Different types of HRT

There are more than 50 preparations of HRT licensed for use in the UK. In addition, there are a variety of manufacturing processes that can be used to produce HRT. Oestrogen is available in what are usually called 'synthetic' or 'natural' preparations. Synthetic preparations are made entirely from the chemical reproduction of oestrogen, whereas natural oestrogens, although also chemically synthesised, are reproduced from soya beans or yams. However, conjugated equine oestrogens, which are also considered to be 'natural', are manufactured using the urine from pregnant mares. Progestogens are almost always synthetic, although their structure is derived from plant sources.

Oestrogen

Oestrogen has been shown to be beneficial for the relief of menopausal symptoms such as hot flushes, night sweats, depressed mood, urinary symptoms and vaginal symptoms. It has also been found to be effective for the treatment and prevention of osteoporosis (brittle bone disease) and provides some protection against bowel cancer. Studies also suggest that oestrogen may be protective against heart disease and Alzheimer's disease, although research in this area is ongoing. In particular, the possible protective benefits that oestrogen has to offer for the heart have been found to be lost when given in combination with progesterone (see also Chapter 5). However, oestrogen stimulates the growth of the lining of the womb (endometrium), and if this is not subsequently broken down, it may become cancerous. In addition to oestrogen, therefore, women who have not had a hysterectomy need to take progesterone for 10–14 days in the latter half of the cycle, in order to break down the endometrium.

In addition to endometrial cancer, oestrogen therapy has been found to be associated with an increased risk of breast cancer and thrombosis (blood clots). The risks and benefits associated with HRT are discussed in more detail later in this chapter.

Progesterone

Progesterone cannot be given orally as it is rapidly broken down in the gut. It can be absorbed, however, when used in the form of a vaginal cream or pessaries, although this may not be desirable, as they tend to produce copious waxy discharge. Synthetic forms of progesterone, called progestogens, are therefore frequently used. These can be taken either orally in a tablet form, or as an implant or intrauterine (inserted into the womb via a coil), or as a patch applied to the skin.

In addition to being used with oestrogen, progestogens may also be used in isolation as a treatment for irregular and heavy bleeding. Prior to the menopause there may be an absence of ovulation. Without ovulation, the body does not produce progesterone, which often leads to irregular and very heavy bleeding. Progestogens can be given, therefore, over the latter half of the cycle for 10–14 days, so that when the therapy is stopped, lighter menstruation begins.

Irregular and heavy bleeding can also be treated through the insertion of an intrauterine coil, containing a capsule of progestogen (Levonorgestrel). Once the coil (called a Mirena coil) is inserted into the uterus, it will release a continuous low dose of Levonorgestrel for approximately five years. After around three months of use, the majority of women find a significant reduction in menstrual flow, often ceasing to menstruate completely. An additional potential benefit associated with using this form of progestogen is that it also provides contraception.

Although a few studies have shown that progestogens, when taken in large doses, can be effective in relieving menopausal symptoms, women tend to find such large doses hard to tolerate as they often produce symptoms such as fluid retention, muscle aching, and greasy hair and skin. In addition, there is no evidence that progestogens increase bone mass and studies suggest that they increase the risk of heart disease.

Testosterone

Testosterone is a male hormone which, in women, is produced by the ovaries. The production of testosterone is reduced a few years after the menopause. Although not regularly given as part of hormone replacement therapy, testosterone can be useful for women who experience continuing lethargy, tiredness and loss of libido, despite treatment with oestrogen. At present, testosterone can only be prescribed in the form of implants, and these have to be replaced every six months.

Tibolone

Tibolone is a synthetic steroid that has oestrogenic, progestogenic and androgenic effects. In addition to being marketed for its ability to improve mood and enhance libido, tibolone has been shown to be effective in the relief of hot flushes and in preventing bone loss. The potentially protective benefits of tibolone on the heart have not yet been established, although, so far, studies have shown that there are short-term protective benefits to the heart. Tibolone is generally only prescribed for women who are at least one year post-menopausal. This is because women who are still producing significant amounts of oestrogen, as happens during the menopause and shortly after, tend to experience irregular bleeding when taking tibolone. Not only does this irregular bleeding pattern cause problems for women, but it also requires investigation in order to be sure that it is caused by the therapy and is not due to potentially cancerous changes in the lining of the womb.

The main side-effect of tibolone is weight gain and a tendency to bloating. A few women may also notice an increase in the growth of facial hair when switching from oestrogen therapy to tibolone.

SERMs (selective oestrogen receptor modulators)

In addition to HRT, a new class of drugs has emerged called selective oestrogen receptor modulators (SERMs). Although these drugs do not provide relief from menopausal symptoms, they have been shown to provide significant protection against osteoporosis. The potential protective benefit of SERMs on the heart is currently being investigated. Examples of SERMs are Tamoxifen and Raloxifene. Unlike HRT, SERMs work by stimulating oestrogen receptors in selected tissue sites. Therefore, where oestrogen activation is undesirable, for example in the breasts and the uterus, the receptors are left inactive. When taken on a long-term basis, SERMs should not increase the risk of breast cancer. Research is ongoing in this area.

Hot flushes and leg cramps are regularly reported side-effects associated with SERMs and they are therefore of little benefit to women experiencing menopausal symptoms. As with HRT, a further side-effect of SERMs is the slight increased risk of thrombosis (blood clots).

Do most women take HRT?

By the age of 50 years, almost half of the women in Britain will have tried hormone replacement therapy. Although it first became available in the 1930s, up until recently relatively few women actually took the therapy. Over the past decade, however, the number of women taking hormone therapy has risen steeply. In the *Women's Health Study* survey, 60 per cent of women had tried HRT, although only 42 per cent were still taking it at the time of the survey.

Why do women take HRT?

The survey showed that the most popular reason for taking HRT was for the relief of hot flushes and night sweats. As Figure 8.1 shows, in addition to taking HRT for symptom relief, many women also took the therapy to reduce their risk of osteoporosis. When asked to rank these reasons for HRT use in order of importance,

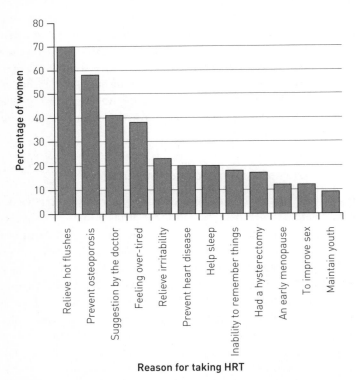

Figure 8.1. Reasons why women take HRT – results from the *Women's Health Study* survey.

however, women indicated that they were taking HRT primarily for the relief of menopausal symptoms, but were glad to have the possible 'added' benefits of protection for the bones. Other key reasons for taking HRT were, advice from the doctor, and because of feeling over-tired.

In addition to the reasons illustrated in Figure 8.1, some women stated that they took HRT for reasons such as dizziness and palpitations, and to improve urinary health. However, these reasons were mentioned by less than 1 per cent of women.

Why do women choose not to take HRT?

Although over half of the women surveyed took HRT, there were many women who chose not to take the therapy. Reasons for this varied. As Figure 8.2 shows, and it is probably not surprising, the most popular reason for not taking HRT is a lack of perceived need for the therapy. Other frequently cited reasons were the belief that the menopause was natural, a fear of cancer, and also a general dislike of taking medicines.

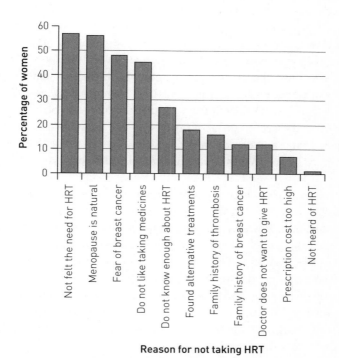

Figure 8.2. Reasons why women do not take HRT – results from the *Women's Health Study* survey.

Which type of HRT?

If you have decided to take HRT, the type that you will be prescribed will depend upon (1) whether you have had a hysterectomy or not, and (2) whether you are at the start or middle of the menopause, or have passed it.

Women who have had a hysterectomy only require oestrogen therapy, as they do not need progesterone to protect the lining of the womb against cancer. An oestrogen implant is often offered at the time that women have their hysterectomy. Following surgery, however, women may either continue with implants, or they may be advised to switch to an alternative form of oestrogen.

Women who have not had a hysterectomy need to take progesterone in order to reduce the risk of endometrial cancer (cancer of the lining of the womb). As discussed in Chapter 3, women may opt to have an endometrial ablation/resection rather than a hysterectomy. If wanting to take HRT, however, women who have had an endometrial ablation/resection will still need to take progesterone as there are often small patches of endometrial tissue left behind, which may become stimulated by oestrogen therapy.

During the menopause, progestogens can either be given for the last 10–14 days of each 28-day cycle, or a 3-monthly cycle treatment may be used, where oestrogen is given for 70 days, followed by 14 days of combined oestrogen and progesterone and then 7 days of neither oestrogen nor progesterone. The advantage of the 3-monthly treatment cycle is that women only have to have a bleed every 3 months as opposed to monthly. However, some women find that they experience erratic bleeding on the 3-monthly regimes and they may therefore be better sticking with the monthly treatment. Unfortunately, women often report side-effects with progestogens, in particular headaches, bloating, weight gain, acne, and depression or mood swings. Some of these side-effects, however, may be reduced or eliminated when a different type of progestogen is taken.

When women are at least 1 year past the menopause, they may wish to take both oestrogen and progesterone continuously every day as this should eliminate bleeding altogether. However, these preparations are generally only given once women reach the age of 54 years, as this is the age by which 80% of women will be post-menopausal (1 year after the cessation of menstruation). Women who take these continuous preparations before they are post-menopausal are very likely to experience irregular bleeding. The 'no-bleed' preparations often cause bleeding problems in the first few months of use, with some women reporting continuous spotting. Around three-quarters of women, however, will be able to achieve 'no-bleed' within 6 months of use.

Different ways of taking HRT

Tablets

Tablets are the most frequently prescribed form of HRT, although there are many different types and they are manufactured by a number of different pharmaceutical companies. They usually come in 28-day packs, with some providing a combination of oestrogen and progestogen in one tablet, and others being delivered separately.

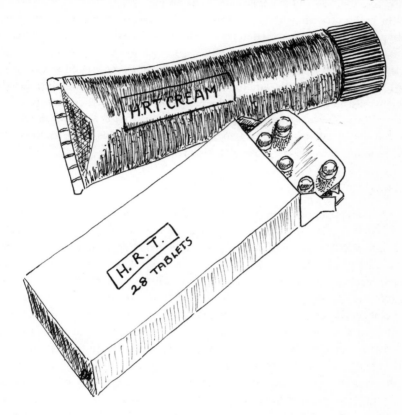

Implants

Oestrogen and progestogens can be taken in the form of an implant, where a small pellet, slightly smaller than a pea, is inserted into the fatty tissue of the skin. The most popularly used sites of insertion are the abdomen or the thigh, as these areas tend to have a large supply of fatty tissue. Women who have had a hysterectomy often prefer implants because they do not have to remember to take the therapy each day. Women who have not had a hysterectomy, however, still have to take progesterone tablets or patches for 10 to 14 days in every 28-day cycle. If progestogens are taken continuously, they can be given via an implant.

Implants are generally replaced every 4 to 6 months. However, they are difficult to remove and so the old implant is usually left under the skin and the new one placed in a slightly different site. Your family doctor may be able to insert your implant, although many general practitioners are not trained in this procedure and so you may have it have this done at the hospital.

The major problem with implants is that women can experience what is called 'tachyphylaxis'. This occurs when very high levels of oestrogen are achieved soon after the implant is inserted. Women then get used to living with much higher levels of oestrogen than normal, and so when the blood oestrogen levels start to drop to more normal levels, symptoms re-appear. Hence women suffering with this problem return to the doctor to have their implant replaced in increasingly shorter spaces of time. Instead of needing a new implant every four to six months, they can find that they need one after just two or three months. If this happens, the doctor may recommend a different route for taking HRT.

Patches

Some women prefer not to take tablets and therefore feel happier taking oestrogen via a patch applied to the skin (transdermal). In addition, there are certain conditions when it is preferable to give oestrogen via this route as it avoids initial breakdown by the liver. This is discussed in more detail later in this chapter. Progestogens are also available in transdermal form. Since reliable absorption of progestogens cannot be achieved through the skin, however, norethisterone is used as it gets broken down into progesterone within the body.

Most women will bleed towards the end of the combined oestrogen and progesterone therapy. However, the first oestrogen patch of the new cycle should still be applied, irrespective of the duration of bleeding.

Patches should be applied to clean, dry skin, in an area where minimal wrinkling occurs on movement. The use of creams or lotions around the site should be avoided, as this will reduce the adhesive properties of the patch. Many women find that the buttocks or the hip are ideal sites. Most patches are designed to be changed every three to four days, although there are now some patches that last for one week. It is necessary, therefore, to check the instructions on the package. In order to minimise skin irritation, the site should be altered when the patch is changed.

Gels

Oestrogen gels are becoming more popular with women, and have become the most frequently used form of HRT by women in France. One of the key reasons that women like using HRT gels is that they make it possible to find the most suitable dose of oestrogen for each individual woman. They also allow women to use the lowest dose possible for symptom relief. These lower dose levels, however, are unlikely to provide protection against osteoporosis. The dose of oestrogen should be altered with guidance from the doctor. A further advantage of oestrogen gels is that they are less likely than patches to cause a skin reaction.

Vaginal preparations

Creams, pessaries and rings containing oestrogen may be applied directly to the vagina to alleviate vaginal dryness and urinary symptoms such as frequency in passing urine and recurrent urinary infections. These preparations contain oestrogen (e.g. Premarin, Vagifem) or oestriol (e.g. Ovestin, Ortho-Gynest), a broken down product of oestrogen. Preparations containing oestriol target specific receptors in the vagina and do not have any effect on other symptoms such as hot flushes. In addition, since oestriol receptors are only present in the vagina, treatment does not stimulate the endometrium (lining of the womb). Women taking oestriol preparations are therefore not exposed to an increased risk of endometrial cancer and do not need to take progesterone replacement.

Preparations containing oestrogen target oestrogen receptors throughout the body. However, very small quantities are absorbed into the bloodstream and it is unlikely that this will be enough to relieve symptoms such as hot flushes. Women are generally advised to use oestrogen cream daily for a couple of weeks, followed by once- or twice-weekly treatments. If taken in this way, progesterone is generally not necessary as the dose is not high enough to stimulate the endometrium.

Nasal spray

Recent developments have led to oestrogen therapy being available in a nasal spray, where one spray is inserted into each nostril each day. As with oestrogen gels, the dose can be altered slightly so that the lowest possible dose can be used. Lower doses, however, are unlikely to provide protection against osteoporosis. Women who have not had a hysterectomy will also need to take progesterone.

How long should I take HRT for?

In the past, women have taken HRT for relatively short periods of time, with many studies showing that the therapy was being discontinued within the first year or two of use. Side-effects of the therapy, such as bleeding problems, headaches and fluid retention, were frequently cited reasons for women stopping the therapy.

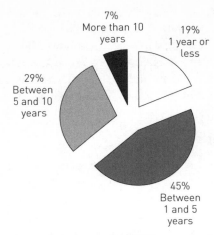

Figure 8.3. Length of time that women take HRT – results from the *Women's Health Study* survey.

Developments in HRT, however, have meant that women tend to tolerate the therapy more easily. This, coupled with an increased focus on disease prevention, has led to an increased duration in the use of HRT.

As Figure 8.3 shows, the *Women's Health Study* survey revealed that almost a third of women had taken HRT for five to ten years, with 7% of women taking the therapy for more than 10 years.

The length of time that HRT is taken for is largely dependent upon the reasons for taking the therapy in the first place. If it is being taken for symptom relief, then it may only be required for a couple of years. If HRT is being taken for the prevention of osteoporosis, it needs to be taken for a much longer period of time. This longer use of the therapy, however, may increase the risk of conditions such as breast cancer.

What are the risks associated with HRT?

With a shift towards the long-term use of HRT, there has been an increased reporting of complications associated with the therapy. However, as discussed at the start of this book, largely due to differences in study design and types and dosages of HRT, conflicting messages about the benefits and risks associated with the therapy have been reported. Indeed, ongoing research means that new discoveries continue to emerge, which lead to further changes in what we understand to be the pros and cons of HRT. This often leaves women confused about whether to commence the therapy or remain on it. Having already discussed the benefits of taking HRT for symptom relief in Chapter 2, and for disease prevention in this chapter and in Chapter 5, the risks will now be outlined.

Breast cancer

One in every nine women in the UK will develop breast cancer.

In the past, there has been a great deal of controversy surrounding the association between HRT and breast cancer, with some studies reporting oestrogen to be protective against the disease and others reporting an increased risk. A study published in 1997, however, used data collected in 51 different studies, and was able to show that the chances of a woman getting breast cancer increased by 2.3 per cent each year in women taking HRT.

An even more recent study of HRT (Women's Health Initiative) reported similar findings in 2002, in that the longer the time that women took HRT for (continuous oestrogen and a form of progesterone), the greater their risk of breast cancer. This very large study of over 16 000 women showed that after 4 years of HRT use, women started to be at an increased risk of breast cancer, compared to women who did not take the therapy. The actual size of increased risk was, however, like the previous study, fairly low. For every 10 000 women taking HRT, eight more will develop breast cancer each year, compared with 10 000 women not taking the therapy. Although the study was stopped after 5 years (because of the increased risk of breast cancer), the results showed that the chances of developing breast cancer when taking HRT increased the longer the therapy was taken for. A second arm of this study, using oestrogen only, is ongoing, with results expected in 2005.

Heart problems

Although studies have shown that the prolonged use of oestrogen is protective against heart disease, progesterone has been shown to significantly reduce the beneficial effects of oestrogen on the heart. Indeed, the Women's Health Initiative study described above showed that for every 10 000 women taking oestrogen and progesterone, seven more will have a heart attack each year, compared with women not taking the therapy. The effect of oestrogen alone on the heart remains unclear.

Thrombosis

In addition to the risk of breast cancer, like the contraceptive pill, HRT has been found to carry an increased risk of thrombosis (blood clots), with the excess risk being greatest during the first year of use. This increased risk is again, fairly small, with studies showing that for every 10 000 women taking HRT, eight more will develop a thrombosis each year, compared with 10 000 women not taking HRT. After this first year of HRT use, the risk of thrombosis appears to go down, and may be reduced to the same level as women who are not taking the therapy.

Strokes

The Women's Health Initiative study on HRT, mentioned above, found that, in addition to an increased risk of breast cancer, thrombosis and heart disease, women taking continuous oestrogen and a form of progesterone are at an increased risk of having a stroke compared to women not taking the therapy. Again, the risk is fairly small, and for every 10 000 women taking HRT, eight more will have a stroke each year, compared with women not taking the therapy. As discussed in Chapter 1, the body's oestrogen appears to be protective against strokes and so it may be possible that oestrogen therapy (as opposed to a combination of oestrogen and progesterone) will help reduce the occurrence of strokes. Further research into this is currently being carried out.

Endometrial cancer (cancer of the lining of the womb)

During the 1970s a number of studies showed that women taking oestrogen therapy had up to a sevenfold increase in the risk of endometrial cancer, depending on the dose and duration of oestrogen use. With the addition of progestogens, however, either continuously or for the latter half of the cycle, the risk of endometrial cancer is significantly reduced. Nevertheless, studies suggest that whilst the additional use of progestogens with oestrogen therapy does eliminate some of the increased risk of endometrial cancer, it is not necessarily totally eliminated, particularly when oestrogen is taken on a long-term basis (over 5 years). Where progestogens are taken continuously with oestrogen, studies have shown that there is no increased risk of endometrial cancer.

High blood pressure

Although HRT does not usually cause a rise in blood pressure, there have been reports of a few women experiencing a sudden rise in blood pressure after com-mencing HRT. It is, therefore, advisable to have your blood pressure checked three months after starting HRT. Following this, blood pressure measurements are usually only carried out as part of a general health check.

Gallstones

Studies have shown that women taking HRT are at a slight increased risk of stones developing in the gall bladder. Reports have shown that for every 185 women treated with HRT, one additional woman each year will have gall bladder surgery, compared with women not taking the therapy.

Contra-indications to hormone replacement therapy

As with most therapeutic drugs, there are certain circumstances in which HRT should not be taken. HRT should not be taken if a woman:

- Has an active venous thrombosis (clot in the leg).
- Has severe liver disease.
- Has recurrent breast cancer.
- Has recurrent endometrial (lining of the womb) cancer.
- Is pregnant.

In addition to these conditions, there are a number of other circumstances where women should be medically investigated prior to commencing HRT:

- Abnormal vaginal bleeding.
- A breast lump.
- Previous breast cancer.
- Strong family history of breast cancer.
- Previous endometrial cancer.
- Previous venous thrombosis (clot in the leg).
- Strong family history of venous thrombosis.

The following conditions might also be affected by HRT and therefore may need further consideration prior to commencing the therapy:

Gallstones

Women who have got gallstones may be better suited to taking HRT patches as opposed to tablets, as oestrogen, when absorbed through the skin, is not initially broken down by the liver.

Previous liver disease

Women who have had previous liver disease should have liver function tests carried out before commencing HRT. Use of a non-oral HRT (for example, patches) would be preferable, as these preparations are not initially broken down in the liver.

Diabetes

HRT may decrease glucose intolerance and therefore women with diabetes will need to monitor their glucose levels more carefully when starting HRT.

Endometriosis

Women who have been diagnosed as having endometriosis are generally able to take HRT, although they are often advised to take oestrogen (with the addition of progesterone if they have not had a hysterectomy) continuously. The reason for continuous use of oestrogen and progesterone, even in women under the age of 54 years, is that the endometriosis appears to be worse when there are swings in oestrogen levels. Thus, it has been suggested that it is not so much the level of oestrogen that makes endometriosis worse, but rather that it gets worse when the oestrogen levels fall and then rise again. However, women under the age of 54 years who have not had a hysterectomy may get problems with irregular bleeding.

Fibroids

Fibroids will reduce in size after the menopause because they are no longer being stimulated by oestrogen. Women who have fibroids, however, may find that HRT causes them to re-grow.

Migraine

Women who suffer from migraines will either improve with HRT or get worse. Some women find that one brand of HRT is better at reducing migraines than others. There is no means, however, of telling which women will experience improvements in migraine when taking HRT. It often has to be left to trial and error.

High blood pressure

Most studies indicate that HRT has little effect on blood pressure and therefore having high blood pressure should not be a contra-indication to taking HRT.

Varicose veins

Women with varicose veins have an increased risk of venous thrombosis (clots in the legs), particularly after surgery. Therefore, HRT may not be advisable for women with varicose veins who are undergoing surgery.

Epilepsy

Some anti-epileptic drugs stimulate the liver to produce substances that reduce the effectiveness of HRT. It is therefore preferable to use non-oral preparations of HRT that are not initially broken down by the liver.

Systemic lupus erythematosis

This autoimmune disease may deteriorate when HRT is taken.

Heart attack

A recent study has shown that women with heart disease were at risk of suffering further heart problems during the first year of taking HRT. Following this first year of use, HRT was shown to provide some protective benefits for the heart in women who already had heart disease.

Should I take HRT?

Many women find it difficult to decide whether they should take HRT or not, and as can be seen in many chapters of this book, the decision is made more complex by virtue of the fact that much still has to be discovered about the therapy. Nevertheless, by considering the pros and cons surrounding HRT, it is possible to reach an informed decision.

Weighing up the pros of HRT you might want to think about the following:

- Relief of menopausal symptoms. Ask yourself how bad your symptoms are and in what ways do they interfere with your quality of life? Are there any changes that you can make in your lifestyle that may make symptoms less severe? (See Chapter 2.)

- Bone protection. Are you at high risk of osteoporosis? If not, can you make lifestyle changes that will reduce your risk of osteoporosis? (See Chapter 5.) If you do have a high risk of osteoporosis, or have been diagnosed as having osteoporosis, you may wish to consider taking HRT. Five fewer women each year, in every 10 000 women, will get a hip fracture because they take HRT.

- Heart protection. Are you at high risk of heart disease? If not, can you make lifestyle changes that will reduce your risk of heart disease? (See Chapter 5.) If you do have a high risk of heart disease AND have had a hysterectomy, you may wish to consider oestrogen therapy. If you have not had a hysterectomy, and therefore need to take progesterone, HRT is likely to *increase* rather than reduce your risk of heart problems.

In addition, HRT has been found to reduce the chances of having bowel cancer, with six fewer women each year, in every 10 000 women, getting bowel cancer when taking HRT, when compared to women not taking the therapy.

Having considered your need for HRT, you now need to weigh this up against the following possible risks associated with HRT:

- Breast cancer. An additional eight women each year, in every 10 000 women, will develop breast cancer if they take HRT for over 5 years.

- Thrombosis (blood clots) especially in the first year of use. An additional eight women each year, in every 10 000 women, will develop a thrombosis when taking HRT.

- Endometrial (lining of the womb) cancer with long-term use. There is probably a small increased risk of endometrial cancer, especially when progesterone is taken cyclically, and when HRT is taken for more than 5 years.

- Unpleasant side-effects from HRT. Side-effects may or may not occur.

What should I do if I want to stop HRT?

There are many reasons why women decide to stop taking HRT. In the *Women's Health Study* survey, some women stated that HRT did not have the desired effect on symptoms and therefore they saw little point in continuing with it. Others wished to stop taking the therapy in order to check whether they were still having menopausal symptoms and, therefore, whether the therapy was still necessary. Concern over the possible long-term effects of taking HRT was a further reason for stopping the therapy. The majority of women who stopped taking HRT, however, did so because they found that they were experiencing side-effects. The most frequently reported side-effects were weight gain, headaches and problems with bleeding. Other less frequently reported problems were mood swings, painful breasts, bloating and skin irritation (from patches). Although studies have consistently shown that HRT does not increase body weight, many women reported this to be a key reason for stopping the therapy.

If you have decided to discontinue HRT, you might find it helpful to discuss your decision with your doctor, especially if your reasons for discontinuing the therapy are related to side-effects. There are many different types of HRT and trying a different type, or route of delivery, may help. Ultimately, however, the decision to stop taking HRT is yours, but you may find it helpful to discuss this with your doctor.

When stopping HRT, it is advisable to reduce the dose over a period of time, rather than stopping it abruptly. This will minimise the swings in oestrogen levels, and therefore reduce the incidence of hot flushes, which may be experienced when stopping HRT. When reducing oestrogen doses, however, progesterone (in women who have not had a hysterectomy) should be continued at the same dose to ensure that the lining of the womb remains protected.

Summary

- There are many different forms of HRT. Women who have had a hysterectomy only need to take oestrogen. Those who have not had a hysterectomy, however, need to take a form of progesterone in order to reduce the risk of endometrial cancer (cancer of the lining of the womb). Up until the age of 54 years, women are prescribed progesterone for the latter half of the cycle only. After the age of 54 years, women may take progesterone continuously, in an attempt to eliminate the monthly bleed. Women experiencing continued lethargy and loss of libido, despite treatment with oestrogen, may also wish to take testosterone.

- HRT may be taken as a tablet, an implant, a transdermal patch, a cream, a pessary, a gel and a nasal spray. The choice of route will depend on personal preference and medical history.

- Over half of women in their fifties take HRT, although many stop taking the therapy after 2 or 3 years.

- Women taking continuous oestrogen and a form of progesterone have been found to have a slightly increased risk of breast cancer, heart disease, stroke, and blood clots. They also have a slight decrease in the risk of osteoporosis and bowel cancer.

Contraception after the age of 40

9

From the age of 30 years onwards fertility starts to decline so that, by the age of 40, women have a 20 per cent less chance of getting pregnant than when they were in their twenties. Nevertheless, a substantial number of women in their forties will become pregnant. Official statistics show that every year around 1000 women in the UK become pregnant between the ages of 45 and 49.

Although the menopause does represent the end of fertility, women do not suddenly become menopausal but, as discussed in Chapter 1, hormone levels fluctuate. This can result in an absence of periods for a number of months, followed by a bleed and normal hormone levels, when pregnancy can occur. Because of these fluctuating hormones, women who stop menstruating under the age of 50 are advised to continue using contraception for 2 years after their last period, and women who stop menstruating after the age of 50 should continue using contraception for 1 year after their last period.

There are a number of contraceptive options available for women, some of which may have additional benefits in relieving other symptoms such as irregular or heavy bleeding.

Hormonal preparations

Both oestrogen and progestogens, in large enough doses, are effective contraceptives. Oestrogen works by preventing ovulation and progestogens work by changing the mucus covering the cervix to discourage sperm entry, and by altering the endometrium so that implantation cannot take place. Although hormone replacement therapy contains oestrogen and progestogens, the dose of hormones used is too low to provide contraception.

Low dose combined contraceptive pill

Low dose combined oral contraceptive pills contain both progestogens and oestrogen. Although this form of contraception may be used up until the time of the menopause, owing to the amount of oestrogen required to suppress ovulation and, therefore, provide contraception, its use is associated with an increased risk of venous thrombosis (blood clot). Doctors may, therefore, be reluctant to prescribe it for women who smoke, who are overweight or who are inactive.

The advantage of the low dose combined pill is that the oestrogen intake means that women will experience fewer menopausal symptoms, although these may be marked during the 'pill-free' period when oestrogen levels fall. Heavy and irregular bleeding, often experienced during the years before menopause, is also drastically reduced when taking the combined pill. In addition, the high levels of oestrogen provide protection against bone loss.

Once women reach the age of 50 years, the combined pill can be stopped to determine whether the menopause has been reached. Recent guidelines suggest that the combined pill is safe until after the menopause and, therefore, women may wish to delay stopping it until they are 52–54. Eighty per cent of women will reach the menopause by the age of 54 years and, therefore, women stopping the combined pill may wish to use a barrier method of contraception to be absolutely sure that they will not conceive.

The mini pill

The mini pill contains the progestogen, norethisterone, and may be used by women with risk factors for venous thrombosis (i.e. smoking, overweight, inactivity). It works better as fertility is reduced and is, therefore, just as effective as the combined pill in women over the age of 40. The disadvantages of the mini pill are that the dose of progestogen is not high enough to relieve menopausal symptoms, and many women report problems with continual spotting.

Emergency contraception

The morning-after pill is effective for up to 72 hours after intercourse. Recent recommendations suggest that a high-dose progestogen should be used, as this is considered safer than high-dose oestrogens. The treatment is repeated 12 hours after the initial dose.

Progestogen via an intrauterine device

As discussed in Chapter 8, the progestogen, Levonorgestrel, can be slowly delivered directly into the uterus through an intrauterine device (coil). An important advantage of this form of contraception is that the progestogens act directly where they are needed (the lining of the womb) and, therefore, side-effects are usually avoided. In addition, it is very effective in reducing heavy and irregular bleeding, with most women ceasing to menstruate after three months of use. Initial use, however, may result in spotting. The device can be left in place for up to 5 years.

Progestogen by injection or implant

Progestogens can be given via an injection into the muscle every 3 months, and may be useful for women who are unable to take oestrogen and are likely to forget taking a pill every day. It stops ovulation, however, and has been shown to reduce bone density in women taking it over a long period of time. Progestogen-containing implants can also be inserted under the skin to provide anything up to 5 years contraception, depending on the type and dose of progestogen used.

Non-hormonal contraception

There are a number of barrier methods and spermicides available, many of which have been found to be very effective in women over the age of 40. This is not only because fertility is reduced in older women, but also because older women tend to have more experience in using contraception. In addition, non-hormonal intrauterine devices can provide effective contraception.

Intrauterine devices

Intrauterine devices, popularly known as the coil, have to be inserted by a doctor, but may remain in place for up to 5 years. They can be left in for up to 1 year after the menopause, but need to be checked to make sure that the cervix is not getting too tight to allow removal.

Intrauterine devices are 98 per cent effective in achieving contraception. Where the device fails, the pregnancy is often ectopic, where the embryo implants into the fallopian tube.

Condoms

Both male and female condoms are available. Male condoms can be purchased from a variety of high-street shops and are frequently available from machines in public restrooms. They can be purchased already lubricated with a spermicide or with a non-spermicidal lubrication. Effectiveness is high if used properly, although there is a possibility that the condom might split. If this happens, women should consider taking the morning-after pill. Female condoms (Femidom) can also be purchased, although they tend to be mainly available in chemist stores. The Femidom consists of a loose-fitting polyurethane sheath with a flexible ring at one end and a firmer separate ring, which is used to keep the sheath in place around the cervix. The advantage of the Femidom is that it rarely splits. It can, however, be difficult to insert, and some women (and men) find it causes soreness.

Diaphragms and caps

These are dome-shaped devices that are inserted into the vagina to prevent sperm being able to reach the cervix. They are used in conjunction with spermicides and can be inserted a few hours prior to intercourse. They have to be left in position for 6 hours after intercourse. They are 95 per cent effective in achieving contraception.

Sponges

Sponges impregnated with spermicides are inserted into the vagina prior to intercourse. They are 75 per cent effective in achieving contraception.

Natural methods

Natural methods, such as temperature recording and cycle timing, are not very reliable forms of contraception. Prior to the menopause, when hormones can fluctuate and cycles may vary in length, this method of contraception is even more unreliable.

Summary

- Although fertility starts to decline from the age of 30 years onwards, a substantial proportion of women aged 45–49 years get pregnant each year.

- There are many effective contraception options. Women experiencing problems with heavy bleeding may wish to consider taking progesterone via an intrauterine device, as this is usually effective in reducing bleeding as well as providing contraception.

The future

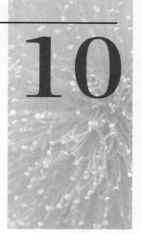

10

Whether you have read this book chapter by chapter, or whether you have chosen to select sections of specific interest, you will have probably noticed that understandings of the menopause are constantly changing.

In addition, the world in which the menopause is experienced has not remained the same, with women's lives taking on quite a different shape to the lives that were experienced in past centuries. Thus, today, the biological changes associated with the menopause often occur at the same time as a number of social changes. Becoming the main carer for elderly relatives, returning to paid employment, and changing relationships with children can all have an impact on a woman's experience of the menopause.

Although the biological changes have probably not altered over time, the ways in which they are dealt with have undergone tremendous change. Moreover, with developments in the pharmaceutical industry, along with a rapid growth in our understanding and use of genetics, things are unlikely to remain constant for too long. Thus, while it might seem strange that back in medieval times the menopause was understood to be due to blood being trapped within the abdomen, in the future, women may be astonished by the twenty-first century experiences of the menopause.

Numerous developments have shown that ovarian tissue can not only be successfully frozen, but also, when implanted at a later date, it can be capable of producing female hormones. Indeed, recent reports of the successful transplantation of an ovary in a Chinese woman with previous ovarian cancer indicate that the future holds many possibilities for women. Whilst this surgery is still very much in its infancy, it suggests that it may be possible, in the future, for women to have ovarian tissue transplanted in order to delay the menopause.

For now, however, if women wish to alter the declining levels of oestrogen associated with the menopause, they have to take it in the form of hormone replacement therapy, or possibly one of the newer phyto-oestrogen products. In addition, drugs that target specific oestrogen-sensitive tissues are now available. Although each of these products plays a part in relieving menopausal symptoms and preventing diseases such as osteoporosis, they all carry with them, possible side-effects. Yet, despite extensive scientific research, the beneficial and harmful effects of oestrogen replacement therapies (including plant oestrogens) are still not fully understood.

Although more work into the use of phyto-oestrogens would be beneficial, there are three large national studies on hormone replacement therapy, each of which will hopefully shed more light on the true value of the therapy:

- The Women's Health Initiative (WHI). This is a study being carried out in the United States to investigate the long-term benefits and risks of oestrogen. The study is due to be completed in 2005. As discussed in Chapter 5, a parallel study testing oestrogen plus progestogen was stopped in 2002, owing to an increased risk of breast cancer in women taking the therapy.

- The Women's International Study of Long Duration Oestrogen after the Menopause (WISDOM) is a British study that aims to determine the long-term risks and benefits of HRT and involves 10 years of treatment with HRT followed by a 10-year follow-up of major health outcomes. The end of the treatment with HRT stage was scheduled for 2009, but following the cessation of the oestrogen PLUS progestogen arm of the WHI trial, the WISDOM study has recently been stopped. Results of data collected so far will be reported over the next year or so.

- The Heart and Estrogen/Progestin Replacement Study (HERS) is another American-based study which started in 1993. The aim of the study is to test the long-term effects of both oestrogen and progestogen on women who have established heart disease. As discussed in Chapter 5, the results of the study so far, have been released, but further data collection continues.

While much of the research focus is on different treatments for the menopause, many women choose not to take any form of treatment. This may be because they do not feel a need for treatment, whether in the form of HRT or a non-hormonal preparations, or it may be because they do not wish to take any of the available therapies. As illustrated in the *Women's Health Study* interviews, the menopause is an individual experience and each woman has her own personal way of facing the experience.

Many women, however, feel the need to consider treatments such as HRT because they are concerned about whether they are at an increased risk of menopause-related disease. In the past, treatments were taken on a short-term basis and were used solely for the relief of menopausal symptoms. This has changed quite markedly within the Western world of today, with women taking HRT for a longer duration, often to help prevent diseases such as osteoporosis. This focus on health risks is a fairly new phenomenon, although one that is growing rapidly. In part, we can understand our heightened concern about health risks as arising because we now enjoy a much longer life expectancy. At birth women can now expect to live to an average of 80 years and men to an average of 75 years. This means, therefore, that women can expect to live at least 30 years of their life after the menopause.

The focus on health risks is also influenced by the increasing availability of medical information. The media frequently report the results of medical studies that illuminate discoveries of the numerous health risks and how these might be decreased by a change in lifestyle or diet, or by taking specific medication. By doing things such as increasing our daily intake of fresh fruit and vegetables, exercising for 20 minutes each day, and reducing our cholesterol intake, we are able to reduce a variety of health risks. These factors, along with many others, not only contribute to a longer life, but also enhance the quality of those extra years. It is not surprising, therefore, that the management of risk has taken on such a high profile. With the ongoing developments in genetics, it is likely that this focus on risk will increase. In the future, therefore, we may find ourselves going to the doctor to get a calculation of our risk profile rather than for treatment for illness.

Summary

- Women's experiences of the menopause have altered over time, with a number of life changes occurring around the same time as the biological changes that are brought about by the menopause.

- There are three key research projects currently under way, the results of which will be released over the next 5 to 10 years.

- Within the Western world today, a focus on health risks encourages us to monitor our health more closely than ever before. For women, this may mean that the menopause signifies a health risk, where diseases such as osteoporosis and heart disease threaten to reduce good health. Alongside these changing views of health risk, medical technology provides a number of treatment options that potentially offer the way to a longer, healthy life. These treatments, however, while bringing a number of benefits, may also create further health risks.

- The menopause is an individual experience and each woman has her own personal way of facing the experience.

Useful addresses

Women's Health

This is a charity that provides a variety of information sources on many aspects of women's health. They have a telephone and postal enquiry service and provide a wide range of leaflets and tapes at a small charge. Available leaflets include:

- Menopause
- Hormone replacement therapy
- Alternative medicine
- Heavy bleeding

Address: 52 Featherstone Street
                  London EC1Y 8RT
Telephone: Helpline 0845 125 5254 (local rate) Mon–Fri 9.30am–1.30pm
Email: womenshealth@pop3.poptel.org.uk
Web address: http://www.womenshealthlondon.org.uk

Women's Health Concern

Women's Health Concern (WHC) is a charity organisation that provides advice and information to women about a number of different health issues. In addition to producing books and leaflets, they provide telephone advice.

Address: PO Box 1629
                  London W8 6AU
Telephone: 020 7938 3932

Amarant Trust

The Amarant Trust is a charitable trust that aims to promote a better understanding of the health problems experienced by mature women and to help prevent and alleviate these problems. Their fee-paying clinic is run from the address below. They have a 24 hour HRT helpline, where you can speak to a nurse: 01293 413 000.

Address: Churchill Clinic
                  80 Lambeth Road
                  London SE1 7PW
Telephone: 020 7401 3855

The National Osteoporosis Society

This is a charity organisation that has been set up specifically to improve the diagnosis, treatment and prevention of osteoporosis. Free telephone advice, along with a number of leaflets on many aspects of osteoporosis are provided. In addition, the society is able to put you in touch with local support groups.

Address:	Camerton
	Bath BA2 0PJ
Telephone:	01761 472 721 (Helpline)
	01761 471 771
Email:	info@nos.org.uk
Website:	www.nos.org.uk

British Heart Foundation

The British Heart Foundation is a charity organisation that aims to play a leading role in the fight against heart disease. In addition to funding research, it provides support and information about the causes, treatment and prevention of heart disease. They provide a number of leaflets and books, which can be ordered directly via their Internet site.

Address:	14 Fitzhardinge Street
	London W1H 6DH
Telephone:	020 7935 0185
Website:	www.bhf.org.uk

Breast Cancer Care

This is a national charity organisation that offers information and support to people affected by breast cancer. The services are free and confidential.

Address:	Kiln House
	210 New Kings Road
	London SW6 4NZ
Email:	bcc@breastcancercare.org.uk
Website:	www.breastcancercare.org.uk
Helpline:	0808 800 6000

Index

John Wiley & Sons

publish a wide range of groundbreaking **books, journals** *and* **online resources**

in many areas...

Also Available in This Series:

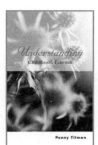
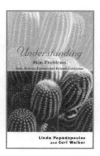
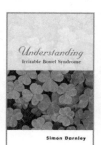
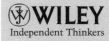